Prevention's

Medical Care Yearbook

1988

Prevention's

Medical Care Yearbook 1988

By the Editors of *Prevention*® Magazine

Edited by Lewis Vaughn,

Assistant Managing Editor, *Prevention*® Magazine

Rodale Press, Emmaus, Pennsylvania

Chapter 5, "Modern Medicine against Stroke," was adapted from *Stroke* (Washington D.C.: U.S. Department of Health and Human Services, 1983).

Chapter 10, "How to Read the Warning Signs on Your Skin," was adapted from *Beauty Is Skin Deep*, by Howard Donsky, M.D. (Emmaus, Pa.: Rodale Press, 1985). Reprinted by permission of the author.

Chapter 12, "Stopping the Hurt of Headaches," was adapted from *Headache: Hope through Research* (Washington, D.C.: U.S. Department of Health and Human Services, 1984).

Chapter 19, "Fighting High Blood Pressure with Modern Medicines," was adapted from *Managing Hypertension*, by James V. Warren, M.D., and Genell J. Subak-Sharpe (Garden City, N.Y.: Doubleday, 1986). Reprinted by permission of the publisher.

Chapter 33, "What to Do about Breast Lumps," was adapted from *My Body, My Decision!* by Lindsay R. Curtis, M.D., Glade B. Curtis, M.D., and Mary K. Beard, M.D. (Tucson, Ariz.: The Body Press—HP Books, 1982). Reprinted by permission of the publisher.

The following chapters were adapted from and reprinted by permission of *Medical Self-Care* magazine, P.O. Box 1000, Pt. Reyes, CA 94956 (free sample magazine available on request): Chapter 24, "The Modern War on Baldness" (May–June, 1987); Chapter 26, "Science against Scars" (March–April, 1987); Chapter 29, "Fighting Back against Prostate Trouble" (July–August, 1986); and Chapter 32, "Is Cervical Cancer Sexually Transmitted?" (September–October, 1986).

Printed in the United States of America on recycled paper containing a high percentage of de-inked fiber.

ISBN 0–87857–748–3 hardcover

2 4 6 8 10 9 7 5 3 1 hardcover

Notice

This book is intended as a reference volume only, not as a medical manual or guide to self-treatment. If you suspect that you have a medical problem, we urge you to seek competent medical help. Keep in mind that nutrition and health needs vary from person to person, depending on age, sex, health status and total diet. The information here is intended to help you make informed decisions about your health, not as a substitute for any treatment that may have been prescribed by your doctor.

Contributors to the *Medical Care Yearbook*

EDITORIAL DIRECTOR: Mark Bricklin, Executive Editor, *Prevention*® Magazine

COMPILER AND EDITOR: Lewis Vaughn, Assistant Managing Editor, *Prevention*® Magazine

CONTRIBUTORS: Stefan Bechtel, Martha Capwell, Michael Castleman, Howard Donsky, M.D., Penelope Kuhn, Gale Maleskey, Michael McGrath, Jeff Meade, Tom Shealey, Lewis Vaughn, Susan Zarrow

EDITORIAL/PRODUCTION COORDINATOR: Jane Sherman

DESIGNER: Glen Burris

COPY EDITOR: Dolores Plikaitis

ASSOCIATE RESEARCH CHIEF, *PREVENTION*® MAGAZINE HEALTH BOOKS: Susan A. Nastasee

ASSISTANT RESEARCH CHIEF, *PREVENTION*® MAGAZINE HEALTH BOOKS: Holly Clemson

RESEARCH ASSOCIATE: Karen Feridun

OFFICE MANAGER: Roberta Mulliner

OFFICE PERSONNEL: Kelly Trumbauer, Kim Mohr

Contents

Introduction
How to Keep Up with Medicine xvii

Part I
Health-Saving Advances

Chapter 1
New Ways to Counter Heart Disease............ 1
A review of five research developments that may change—and improve—the tests and treatments for heart and blood problems. Includes new wrinkles in the diagnosis of symptomless heart disease through ultrasound, cholesterol testing and the treadmill exercise test.

Chapter 2
New Frontiers in Arthritis Relief 5
An update on how arthritics can beat the pain and lead normal lives, with the latest medical news on exercise, food sensitivities, new oral gold-salt medications and the pain-fighting power of positive thinking.

Chapter 3
State-of-the-Art Pain Relief.................... 10
Information from America's top pain clinics on how to halt the hurt, including sensible advice on the surgery option, dealing with depression, TENS therapy, using medications effectively, relaxation techniques, painkilling imagery and more. Also, information on how to find a good pain clinic.

Part II
Progress in Surgery

Part III
New Hope with Better Drug Treatments

Part VII
Women's Health Newsfront

Part VIII
Better Ways to Beat Everyday Health Problems

INTRODUCTION
How to Keep Up with Medicine

You're reading the newspaper, and there on page 32, almost crowded off the page by ads for panty hose and steel-belted radials, is a little news item about a medical advance that ten of your friends and relatives should know about—and that you *certainly* want to know about.

But you almost missed it—and you've probably already missed a lot of other important medical news because it's often so inaccessible. Sometimes the best medical news doesn't get big headlines, or its implications are poorly explained, or it just never filters down to you from the medical journals and research centers.

You're now holding in your hand a modest remedy to this problem—*Prevention's Medical Care Yearbook 1988.*

It's designed to do two things for you. The first: to give you a year's worth of the medical world's most important news . . . the breakthroughs, innovations and insights with the biggest possible impact on your health. The second: to tell you precisely what the information means to you and your family, what doctors have to say about it and how you can use it to make informed decisions about your health.

So the emphasis here is on medical matters that matter—not on super-sophisticated medical gadgets that can help only ten people nor on scientific developments that may have relevance to human health in the year 2010.

Yes, the *Medical Care Yearbook* does cover high-tech medical advances, but generally only those that you can take advantage of today. Laser surgery for the heart, corneal implants, vasectomy-reversal microsurgery, on-the-skin drug patches, state-of-the-art allergy tests, "miracle" drugs, new devices and treatments for impotence—you'll find chapters on these and many other bright ideas in medical technology.

But there's more to modern medicine than high tech. There have also been innovations in low tech and no tech—where treatments work without medical hardware or sophisticated techniques—and this book tells you about them: arthritis therapies, techniques for pain relief, a possible ulcer cure found in your own medicine cabinet, up-to-the-minute advice on avoiding allergy triggers, current tips on lifesaving first aid, and many more.

I'm betting that most of the information in the *Medical Care Yearbook* will be new to you . . . that 90 percent of it relates to someone you know, maybe even someone in your family . . . that 50 percent applies directly to your own health . . . that 10 percent may turn out to be the most important health news you've read in years.

So enjoy—and benefit from—*Prevention's Medical Care Yearbook 1988.*

Lewis Vaughn
Assistant Managing Editor
Prevention® Magazine

PART I:
HEALTH-SAVING ADVANCES

CHAPTER 1
New Ways to Counter Heart Disease

Here are five research developments that may change—and improve—the tests and treatments for heart and blood problems.

Heart disease is still the nation's top killer, but every year science learns more about how to fight it. Here is some important advice from the scientific war front.

Don't Wait for Chest Pains to Warn You

If you think you're relatively safe from a heart attack because you have no symptoms, think again: A recent long-term study found that silent ischemia, a symptomless heart disease, is both riskier and more likely to bring on a heart attack than heart disease accompanied by preliminary chest pains. Ischemia is a blood deficiency in part of the heart's muscle. The flow of blood to that area of the heart tissue may be blocked due to spasms or obstruction of the arteries.

And who should get diagnostic tests to make sure they're not at risk for this silent killer? "Middle-aged men who smoke, who have a family history of high cholesterol and blood pressure or who have diabetes," according to Peter F. Cohn, M.D., of the Health Sciences Center of the State University of New York, Stony Brook, who reported on another study of silent ischemia at an American Heart Association annual meeting.

Should You Lie Down during a Cholesterol Test?

That's the latest question about blood-lipid testing, raised by a team of researchers at the Bowman Gray School of Medicine in Winston-Salem, North Carolina, and the Institute for Aerobics Research and the University of Texas Health Science Center, both in Dallas. The team found that the patient's body position affects the concentration of lipids and lipoproteins in the blood. A prone position diluted blood, while standing concentrated it. (That goes for both men and women.) The researchers say that a physician should consider your position during the test—and the length of time you've spent in it—when he or she interprets test results for serum cholesterol and lipids.

Blood Cholesterol Is Seasonal

Your blood cholesterol level will tend to be higher in winter months and lower in the summer, according to results of a decade-long study. The seasonal difference is small but distinct—an average of 7.4 points, reports David J. Gordon, M.D., of the National Heart, Lung and Blood Institute.

You and your physician should know that the slight difference can affect not only your test results but also your dietary attempts to control cholesterol. The American Heart Association recommends a modified diet for people with cholesterol levels of 200 and higher. But Dr. Gordon points out that a patient whose cholesterol level was 240 in the summer could reduce that level to 190 through a low-fat diet, only to find that, in winter, the level would rise to 200, even if he stuck to his diet. (However, he adds, that doesn't mean you should give up on a prescribed low-fat diet—it's still the recommended way to control cholesterol.)

Dr. Gordon doesn't know what causes the seasonal shift, but he says it's not just a matter of staying indoors more in cold weather or chowing down over the holidays. Winter diet and weight changes may account for just 30 percent of the cholesterol increases, he says. And men living in hot southern areas had slightly greater shifts in cholesterol levels during the winter.

Ultrasound for Ultrasure Diagnosis?

You may be familiar with the use of ultrasound to monitor the fetus in pregnant women, but now a pair of University of Minnesota researchers are using an ultrasound probe they developed to get better assessments of coronary damage. This tool may eventually help physicians decide whether you really need heart bypass surgery.

The university reports that as recently as 1982, 170,000 people in the United States underwent coronary bypass surgery—and, in most cases, the operation decision was based on coronary arteriography test results. The test, which could be replaced by the ultrasound process, involves injecting a radiopaque dye into the heart so that x-rays of the arteries can be taken and any blockage can be detected.

Researchers Carl White, M.D., and Robert Wilson, M.D., say their device, which uses a thin catheter to place an ultrasound crystal directly on or in an artery, will keep physicians from underestimating the extent of obstruction in the arteries—a problem they say is common when arteriography alone is used to diagnose the need for bypass surgery.

Clinical trials of the ultrasound probe have been approved and were scheduled to begin on about 400 patients.

Only after that study is complete will the probes be manufactured for wider use.

Walk a Mile on My Treadmill

That's what a man recovering from acute myocardial infarction (AMI) might want to tell his wife to boost her confidence about his ability to resume a normal routine of physical activity, reported Stanford University researchers in the *American Journal of Cardiology.* When 30 patients were given a treadmill exercise test three weeks after AMI occurred (with no clinical complications), the research team compared the reactions of ten wives who didn't observe the test, ten who did watch it and ten who not only watched but also took a walk on the treadmill themselves.

In counseling sessions after the test, all 30 couples were told just how much physical activity—such as walking, jogging and stationary cycling—the patient could expect to do. Wives were asked to describe their perceptions of what their husbands could handle in terms of physical or emotional stressors, including exercise, sexual activity and getting angry, as well as their husbands' overall cardiac capability.

The result: Wives who actually took part in the test gave their husbands significantly higher votes of confidence. Those participating wives were the only ones whose ratings of what their husbands could do (in terms of physical, emotional and cardiac capabilities) matched their husbands' self-assessments.

CHAPTER 2

New Frontiers in Arthritis Relief

Scientists are finding better ways to beat the pain and are helping arthritics lead normal lives.

If you have arthritis, the odds are four to one that you've been to the arthritis underground for an unproven cure, or that you've contributed to the $1 billion spent each year on less-than-scientific means of pain relief—some call them quack cures—that almost always don't work.

It doesn't have to be that way, though. Today, medical science is making it easier for people with arthritis to rid their aching, swollen joints of the pain and discomfort without resorting to such questionable means. As a result, the prognosis for a relatively comfortable life with this incurable disease is better than ever.

A Boston University Medical School study reinforces this optimism. A five-year examination of about 400 people with rheumatoid arthritis showed little effect on their health status. "We checked their physical and psychological deterioration and their pain levels over the years and found only minor changes for the worse," says Lewis Kazis, Sc.D., of the school's Multipurpose Arthritis Center. Half a decade after the study began, most were still leading normal lives, which contradicts some previous notions about progressive decline in the physical and functional status of people with arthritis.

Findings like those from Boston are glad tidings for many of the 37 million people in the United States who suffer from arthritis. Two-thirds of the victims are women, and two of the most common forms of the disease, osteoarthritis and rheumatoid arthritis, strike females about three times as often as males. Of the 1 million people who develop arthritis each year, about 700,000 are women. It's uncertain why females are more susceptible to a disease whose causes are unknown.

Despite the unknowns, more and more hazy areas are becoming clear. Exercise, for instance, has for years been a topic of hot debate. The old school of thought held that no activity was good for inflamed joints, and rest was almost always the prescription. Now there's newer evidence to the contrary. "Our research shows that rest may not be the best approach in many cases, and prolonged rest may do more harm than good," says Marian Minor, a clinical instructor at the University of Missouri-Columbia School of Medicine.

Sixty people aged 21 to 83 with rheumatoid arthritis and osteoarthritis in their legs and feet did deep-water exercises, such as water jogging, and walking on land, working up to 30-minute walks three times a week. "Many of the people had already heard that exercise might help and had tried some type of activity. But they failed to find relief because they attempted exercise that was too strenuous, such as running or aerobic dancing," says Minor.

At the end of 12 weeks, the participants showed improvements in their endurance and aerobic power. There was no worsening of their arthritis, and in some cases a slight improvement was noted.

"The exercise didn't make their arthritis go away," she says. "As they got healthier and stronger and their stamina improved, they felt better, and this took their minds off their arthritis somewhat. The pain assumed a smaller role in their lives. We know from studies that people in pain who sit around all day get depressed, their pain threshold decreases and discomfort dominates their lives.

"The important thing for people with arthritis to remember is that to gain overall fitness, they don't need fast-paced exercises that could harm them. Some form of aerobic activity that works the large muscle groups for about 20 minutes, such as walking or bicycling, is all that's needed."

What about Diet?

Another point of contention in arthritis research has been the effect of diet on the disease. While some scientists suggest that food allergies and fatty foods can aggravate arthritis, others discount the claims as unscientifically based. Results from a Florida investigation now offer additional evidence to support the former.

"Certain rheumatic diseases may indeed be related to sensitivities to particular foods," says Richard Panush, M.D., a rheumatologist at the University of Florida and the Veterans Administration Medical Center in Gainesville. Studies by Dr. Panush are now under way to test that theory.

While he suggests that alterations in diet may benefit some people with a rheumatic disease, Dr. Panush stresses that nutritional therapy is still experimental and that more work is needed to identify food-allergic people with arthritis and determine how effective changes in diet will be.

A Temporary Pain

What may seem like arthritis to some people may actually be transient osteoporosis. The syndrome is similar to regular osteoporosis in that some bone deteriorates, but the transient type is only temporary and is localized in one or two joints. A bout can be successfully treated using aspirin for pain relief. Simple rest helps the bone rebuild itself, so there's no permanent damage.

"It's easy for an aching person to confuse this syndrome with arthritis, because both involve pain of the joints," says rheumatologist Sharad Lakhanpal, M.D., of the Mayo Clinic in Rochester, Minnesota. "The difference is that with transient osteoporosis, there's no inflammation of the joint as there is with arthritis."

The condition is usually found in the hips, legs and ankles, although it can appear in the arms and shoulders. It's slightly more prevalent in males in the 30-to-50 age group, and the cause is unknown. Because the condition comes and goes and is often misdiagnosed, it's uncertain how many people are affected.

Transient osteoporosis, which falls in the rheumatic disease category along with arthritis, can be successfully treated and may pass with no long-term damage. Besides taking aspirin for pain, protecting the affected joint from exertion is important, because the bone is brittle for a while. "The key is to give the joint rest and avoid stressing or shocking the joint when it flares up. It's merely a matter of using common sense and not making any sudden moves that could cause a fracture," says Dr. Lakhanpal.

The Impact of Emotions

Emotions are rapidly becoming recognized as playing an important role in dealing with arthritis pain. Researchers from the Indiana University Multipurpose Arthritis Center in Indianapolis are showing how the mind and a person's will can help overcome discomfort. They phoned elderly people with arthritis every two weeks to check their status and offer encouragement. After six months those people reported less pain and disability, they felt better about themselves, and there was an improvement in their ability to do everyday activities.

One way of maintaining positive self-esteem with a chronic disease is to relate your own condition to others in similar situations. Researchers from the University of Connecticut School of Medicine studied the social comparisons people with rheumatoid arthritis make to help cope.

"The people in our study perceived their diseases as being slightly less severe than average," says psychologist Carol Pfeiffer, Ph.D. "Many felt they could function better than others or thought their disabilities were less visible. They saw themselves as coping better because they tended to dwell less on the negative aspects of having arthritis. We suggest that people try to find some way to make positive comparisons with others in similar situations."

The More You Know

Researchers from Vanderbilt University School of Medicine in Nashville have come up with similar findings about dwelling on the negative. After studying the education level of arthritics, they found that those with more years of education, especially those who attended college, function better and generally feel better than those with less schooling.

"Our observation is that the more educated arthritics don't just sit back and accept their painful fate. They read, they aggressively seek out information about their condition, and they ask questions of their doctors," says Ted Pincus, M.D., of Vanderbilt's Division of Rheumatology and Immunology. "With a chronic disease, such as arthritis, they're treated by a physician, but most of the time they're on their own to reason with the pain day in and day out. Those people who make the extra effort realize that, in most cases, arthritis can be managed, that it isn't as bad as it seems and isn't hopeless. Now we have to find some way to get this message across to the people with arthritis who don't know this."

Golden Relief

When none of the more conventional measures brings relief, injections of gold salts are sometimes an option for treating rheumatoid arthritis. But recently a more convenient oral version has appeared on the market. The three-milligram capsules are available by prescription (the generic name is auranofin), are about as effective as the injections and are said to have fewer serious side effects.

About 125,000 people worldwide have tried oral gold so far. The new form, like the injections, isn't cheap, however. A cost-benefit study by researchers at McMaster University in Hamilton, Ontario, found the average cost for health improvement from oral gold was about $700 after 21 weeks and about $2,000 after a year. Injectable gold costs ran almost $900 for the 21-week period, but about $1,000 for a year's worth of treatments.

Comforting Thoughts

As science continues to dig deeper into the arthritis riddle, more answers will surface, leading investigators and arthritis patients to believe that somewhere there are cures. Perhaps stress plays a role, as University of Virginia researchers recently suggested when they noticed that increased stress meant a worsening of rheumatoid arthritis symptoms. In the meantime, while waiting for more pain-relief breakthroughs, victims can take comfort in the thought that they no longer have to sit and suffer helplessly. Unlike the generation before them, people with arthritis today can, in most cases, control their fate—and their pain.

CHAPTER 3

State-of-the-Art Pain Relief

Here's what top clinics have learned about beating chronic pain.

Most of us are no strangers to pain. We've endured the temporary travail of childbirth, broken bones, sinus headaches or worse.

For some, though, pain becomes something that must be faced every day. It may be generated by backache, arthritis, an old injury, diabetic nerve damage or even terminal cancer.

The pain commandeers our bodies and minds. It restricts our ability to work, to enjoy life, even to think straight. It becomes a terrible tangle of physical and psychological problems that can no longer be solved by simple means.

Some chronic sufferers look to pain-treatment clinics for help. Most are small and offer limited services, such as acupuncture or biofeedback. Some treat only certain disorders, like backache or face and jaw pain. Others are part of major university hospitals or prestigious private clinics, and these offer much more. Their staffs include anesthesiologists, neurologists, psychiatrists and physical and occupational therapists, among others.

These centers try to develop a total program for pain relief that suits each individual. Their approaches vary. Some specialize in medical diagnosis and treatment—drugs or surgery. Others have a psychological orientation, with changes in thinking and behavior their main goals. Some offer exercise and occupational therapy intended to get you back to work. Many others are interdisciplinary and include all three aspects in their treatment.

Some Strategies for Coping

Here is advice from some of these leading centers to the people who have to face pain every day.

Try nonsurgical therapies, and if you do consider further surgery, consider carefully. Many of the people who end up at pain centers have been chewed up and spit out by the medical establishment. They've seen more doctors, had more operations and tried more drugs than they care to count. Nothing has worked. In some cases, medical treatment has made their pain worse.

A major pain center evaluates your medical records and gives you a complete physical exam to see if you might be one of the few who can benefit from further surgery. When it comes to more surgery, though, you might as well know what doctors know—the more operations you have, the less likely another is to be successful.

All surgery can cause new pain by damaging nerves and creating scar tissue. Some treatments, like alcohol injections to deaden peripheral nerves, can cause pain that's very hard to treat.

"With a lot of pain problems there is no agreed-upon treatment, so you have to shop very carefully," says Dennis Turk, Ph.D., director of the Center for Pain Evaluation and Treatment at the University of Pittsburgh Medical School. "I'd tell people to have a workup by a competent orthopedist or physiatrist, a neurologist, whatever specialties are involved, and then to start with the least invasive treatments."

You may find that transcutaneous electrical nerve stimulation (TENS), which uses pocket-size devices that deliver

Shopping for a Pain-Treatment Clinic

The average pain-clinic patient has years of suffering, doctor shopping and at least an operation or two behind him. He's likely to be dependent on painkilling drugs. Needless to say, doctors would prefer to see patients before their pain has become a way of life. (Doctors consider pain "chronic" if it has lasted longer than six months.)

If you think you are a candidate for a pain center, shop carefully. Your success will depend on choosing the one that's right for you. Most major pain clinics require a doctor's referral, and your doctor can help you choose.

Only about 20 pain clinics scattered around the country are truly interdisciplinary, offering more than one method of pain control. Most are associated with large universities. A small number are private. Find out if the center you are considering is interdisciplinary or uses a single approach—diagnostic or rehabilitative, medical or psychological. It will certainly affect the kind of treatment you receive.

Many smaller centers may offer just TENS, acupuncture or nerve blocks. They may be effective if they are dealing with only one particular kind of problem, like headache or backache.

a mild electrical current to the painful area, helps your pain. So may acupuncture or some of the methods discussed below. A nerve block, a common treatment for chronic back pain, can be quite effective in the right hands. "But it should be considered only before the last resort—surgery," says Lee Nauss, M.D., an anesthesiologist with the Mayo Clinic's Pain Center in Rochester, Minnesota.

Choose either an interdisciplinary center or one with an area of specialization that matches your problem. Some centers focus on treating quadriplegics or paraplegics. Some won't treat people in litigation over their injury. Some won't treat cancer patients; others specialize in that area.

It's hard to nail down a clinic's "success rate." Some of the best clinics take on the most hard-core patients, which pulls their success rates down. Then there's the problem of defining success. The people who are paying the costs—insurance companies—most often define it as the ability to return to work. If that is your goal, make sure it's the center's, too. P.R.I.D.E., in Dallas, Texas, specializes in occupational rehabilitation and gets people back to work at a rate that is twice the national average.

Other centers consider themselves successful if their patients leave drug free, with healthier bodies, new optimism, a better understanding of their pain problem and some reduction in pain.

The major pain-treatment centers are quite expensive. Three weeks of inpatient treatment can run to $10,000 and possibly even more. Medical insurance coverage varies tremendously. Most companies pay some, but not all, of the costs.

For self-help information and assistance in choosing a pain center, contact the National Chronic Pain Outreach Association, (703) 368–7357.

"The point is, you can always move on to surgery if you need to, but once you've had surgery, you can't reverse it," Dr. Turk says. "We've had patients come in here in wheelchairs, not because of their original pain but because of surgery they had to relieve that pain."

Even when surgery does work, it often does not provide total relief. People still need other ways to control their pain.

Get medical help for your depression. It's normal for people with chronic pain to become depressed, and it's easy to see why. Their lives have taken a drastic turn for the worse. They may feel helpless, withdrawn and indecisive. They may have sleep and appetite disturbances and crying spells, and they may lose interest in sex.

Doctors initially treated depression to make it easier for people to deal with the psychological problems associated with pain. In the process, they discovered that antidepressants acted as pain relievers by changing the balance of biochemicals in the brain. The drugs increased levels of serotonin, an important neurotransmitter. They also raised levels of endorphins, naturally occurring painkillers in the body. As a result, the perception of pain was lessened.

Bicyclic and tricyclic antidepressants like Elavil and Sinequan are known pain relievers. In a recent National Institutes of Health study, amitriptyline (found in Elavil and several other antidepressants) was found to relieve the pain of diabetic neuropathy, a tough-to-treat ailment. The drug worked well even in people who were not depressed.

See a psychiatrist or other doctor with good experience in treating depression to make sure you get the help you need. Antidepressants are not narcotic and have less harmful side effects than the types of drugs mentioned below.

Get off addictive drugs. One of the first things most pain clinics do is wean their patients from narcotic painkillers, sleeping pills and tranquilizers. Some terminally ill patients, however, continue to need strong medication to relieve pain.

"It's not that these drugs don't work. They do, but for most people they are needed in ever-increasing amounts, and they end up creating many more problems than they solve," says Nelson Hendler, M.D., assistant professor and psychiatric consultant in the Department of Neurosurgery at Johns Hopkins University School of Medicine in Baltimore and director of the Mensana Clinic, a private pain-treatment center in Stevenson, Maryland. "They can decrease memory and intellect, cause depression and irritability and interfere with natural sleep."

These drugs are slowly replaced with biofeedback or other forms of therapy and, occasionally, with nonnarcotic pain relievers like aspirin or ibuprofen.

Stop thinking like a victim. Chronic pain sufferers are often fearful and angry, especially at doctors, and sometimes with good reason. But they also feel dependent and out of control of their situation, and that only makes things worse.

"They give us all the power. They want us to take their pain away," says Robert D. Kerns, Ph.D., an assistant clinical professor at Yale University School of Medicine and coordinator of the pain-management program at the Veterans Administration Medical Center, West Haven, Connecticut.

"We tell them that even though they are coming to a psychologically based program, we believe their pain is real. That is not an issue. What is an issue is that medical technology cannot cure their pain. The relief they are looking for is going to come from a psychological approach. We point out that pain is influenced by many things that are not physical but mental, and those we can deal with."

Basic to his and many other psychologically oriented programs is giving back to patients the power, and the tools, to minimize their own pain, Dr. Kerns says. "We help them develop a lifestyle that lets them once again do things they enjoy—to go back to work, to be a husband and father, to play tennis, to get a good night's sleep."

Learn to relax your pain away. One of the first and most impressive inklings of an individual's power to control his pain comes when he is hooked up to a biofeedback machine, Dr. Turk says.

"We use biofeedback to demonstrate to people the amount of control they have over their bodies," he says.

"During their initial assessment, we show them just how much they can relax their muscles. And we tell them that if they can do this in the laboratory in such a brief period, think what they can do in a relaxed setting with some practice."

Relaxed muscles are important in pain control because pain tends to cause muscle tensing, which leads to further pain, creating an endless cycle. Tense muscles produce more of a chemical irritant, lactic acid. They are more likely to go into spasm and can squeeze off blood flow to an injured area. "There's no doubt that relaxing the muscles in a painful area reduces pain," Dr. Turk says.

The overall relaxation that comes with biofeedback, hypnosis or relaxation training also relieves stress, says Kenneth Greenspan, M.D., director of the Center for Stress and Pain-Related Disorders at Columbia-Presbyterian Medical Center, New York City.

"Stress can add considerably to the perception of pain at the highest levels of the brain," Dr. Greenspan says. "Stress reduces levels of endorphins, painkilling biochemicals that play an important role in our assessment of pain."

If you are looking for ways to relax at home, try relaxation or stress-management tapes or books, available at most bookstores and libraries. Inexpensive biofeedback equipment is also available, although not required.

Get your body moving again. Many people with chronic pain have been inactive for years. Their muscles are weak and their endurance is poor.

"They are afraid to try new activities or activities they have stopped doing because of pain," says Judith Turner, Ph.D., a psychologist with the pain center at the University of Washington. "If they try to do things, their pain increases, and they think they are damaging their bodies, which is usually not the case."

These people become more active than they thought possible, with an individually designed exercise program. "By gradually increasing their level of activity, we can safely get people back to doing lots of things they haven't been able to do for years," Dr. Turner says. "They'll say,

'Yeah, it hurts, but in a good way,'—more like muscle soreness than excruciating pain. Being strong enough to do things for themselves makes people feel really good."

You can devise a similar exercise program to do at home, Dr. Turner says. "Consult a doctor to pick the best exercises for you, start out slow, and set attainable goals," she says. "Even getting out and walking each day is tremendously helpful."

Turn your attention from your pain. Most chronic pain sufferers think of their pain in a strictly physical way, as sensations being created in the nervous system at the site of the pain. In fact, the perception of pain is much more a function of the brain than most people realize. Pain impulses must register in the brain for the pain to be felt.

But what if the brain is too busy elsewhere to focus on incoming pain signals? "We all have ways of distracting ourselves," Dr. Turk says. "We watch TV, read books, go jogging."

We can also imagine. "We show people how they can conjure up certain images and produce a physical response," Dr. Turk says. He'll have people puckering their mouths over an imaginary lemon or moving their eyes back and forth to a tennis match that exists only in their minds. Then he'll have people come up with their own pleasant, positive images they can use to relieve pain.

"Obviously, they are not going to walk around 24 hours a day imagining themselves on a beach in Hawaii," Dr. Turk says. "But when their pain gets bad and there is not much else they can do, they can turn on these images. It's almost like having a TV in your mind."

Get your spouse involved. It's only natural for a husband or wife to try to do what they can for a mate who's hurting. But too often they unknowingly end up helping their mate maintain his or her pain behavior. "When a wife tries to do everything herself and is constantly asking her husband how he feels, she is actually reinforcing his pain," Dr. Kerns says.

"A spouse needs to be attentive and supportive not just when their mate is in pain but especially when he or she is getting out and being more active," says Dr. Turner.

"That's the time to say, 'Gee, I am really happy to see you doing things.' Praise is really important, and something people tend to forget to do."

"Pain patients may say 'I still have pain, but now I can go to work and enjoy going for walks. I don't use medications and I've quit having surgeries.' These things are not to be minimized," Dr. Kerns says. "They'll say their pain

Long-Lasting Pain Relief

Researchers at the University of Illinois in Chicago have encapsulated anesthetic drug particles in microscopic envelopes called microdroplets. Instead of being released into the bloodstream immediately, the drug leaks slowly through the walls of the envelopes, providing sustained relief in the area of the injection. The effects of the anesthetic, methoxyflurane, can last several days with one injection. The longest-acting regional anesthetic currently in use is effective for about four hours. Because methoxyflurane doesn't slow the rate of healing, it can be injected directly into a surgical incision, giving days of sweet relief.

The discovery not only promises relief for pain but also has implications for the whole field of drug treatment. If various drugs can be packaged in a similar way with the same long-term effects, the result could be improved therapies for cancer, inflammatory diseases and other conditions.

The researchers will also look to combine analgesics with other drugs, such as antibiotics and anti-inflammatory drugs, to have multiple effects where needed in a patient's body.

If the new anesthetic proves safe in clinical trials, it may be approved by the U.S. Food and Drug Administration.

sensations are still there, but they are not aware of them. Some people would say if the pain is not being experienced, then indeed it does not exist."

CHAPTER 4

New Techniques for Overcoming Cataracts

Here's how the sight-impairing condition that comes with aging can be corrected surgically and, in some cases, prevented.

Your eyes don't see. Your brain sees. The eyes are merely the collectors of signals that are passed along to the brain for processing into images, much the same way the rooftop antenna receives airwaves that your television turns into pictures.

But in both cases, the reception can become foggy and require adjustment. With the antenna, it could be as simple as shooing the pigeons away. With your eyes, it may mean surgery. In fact, if you're over 40, there's a high likelihood that your slowly fogging vision may be due to cataracts, the third leading cause of blindness and an almost inevitable part of aging. Each year more than 700,000 people develop cataracts, while this year more than a million sight-impaired people will have their cataracts surgically removed.

Not to worry, though, even in the face of such imposing statistics. Cataract surgery has been refined to the point where it's one of the safest operations around, successfully restoring vision 95 percent of the time. More good news: There's even a hint of a possibility that cataracts may be preventable in some cases or, at the least, the loss of vision may be slowed and surgery delayed.

A Gradual Process

The lens of the human eye consists of an outer capsule, or casing, filled with growing lens fibers in layers, almost like an onion. As new fibers form on the outer layers, the older fibers are compressed. This, along with chemical changes that occur naturally during aging and years of exposure to ultraviolet radiation in sunlight, contributes to clouding of the lens, and a cataract is formed. One of every two people over age 40 develops what are called senile cataracts.

The early symptoms are subtle. Colors may seem dull, glare becomes a problem and driving at night is hard because oncoming headlights are momentarily blinding. Eventually sight deteriorates to the point where the world appears as it would if you were walking through heavy fog or clouds.

The cloudy lens cannot be made clear again. In the early stages, you'll probably be able to continue your normal routine, especially if only one eye is affected. In time, the condition will worsen, and you'll have only one choice: surgery. Whether it's one eye or both, no eye exercises, laser treatments or eyedrops will reduce the cloudiness.

The word *cataract* used to make its victims shudder, since it meant surgery and hospitalization for a week or more, part of the time with the head immobilized between sandbags to avoid the slightest jarring. That was followed by a prescription for glasses with lenses as thick as pop-bottle bottoms, or for contact lenses that often weren't well tolerated.

Today, cataract surgery is usually a one-day procedure—barring complications—and you're home for your evening meal. In fact, it has become so routine that many patients approach it too lightly, according to Julius Shulman, M.D., a New York ophthalmologist, who is assistant professor at Mount Sinai Hospital and author of *Cataracts, the Complete Guide—from Diagnosis to Recov-*

ery—for Patients and Families. "Because of the success rate and the fact that it's done on an outpatient basis, people aren't as afraid as they used to be. Too many people take it lightly and don't consider it any more serious than a trip to the dentist. But this is a major eye operation, and it should be approached cautiously after considerable thought. Always keep in mind that it's your decision based on your own symptoms. And don't assume that all eye surgeons are equally qualified, because they're not. Some are better at cornea or retina surgery than cataract surgery."

Complications from surgery, if they develop, usually appear within 24 hours, says Virginia Lubkin, M.D., an ophthalmic surgeon for 40 years, who is attending ophthalmologist at the New York Eye and Ear Infirmary and associate clinical professor at Mount Sinai School of Medicine. "That's the minimum I would like my patients to spend in the hospital, but some insurance programs won't pay for a room overnight."

Fewer Complications

To remove the cataract, surgeons used to routinely perform the intracapsular technique, in which the entire lens—a jellylike core within the rubbery capsule—was removed in one piece. The patient was later fitted with the thick cataract eyeglasses or contact lenses that ride on eye-surface tears.

These days, however, the majority of cataracts are removed with the extracapsular technique. "I've done all of the procedures, but the extracapsular method is the safest because it has the smallest percentage of complications," says Dr. Lubkin.

"It's the method of preference," says David Bogorad, M.D., senior staff ophthalmologist at Henry Ford Hospital in Detroit. "The front part of the capsule is opened, the lens is gently removed and any remaining material is suctioned out. The capsule is left intact, which allows the implant to go behind the iris and more nearly maintains the natural configuration of the eye."

In about 90 percent of the cases, people with cataracts are opting for implants, says Dr. Bogorad. "Unlike contacts and glasses, the implants are maintenance-free."

Implants, or intraocular lenses, are plastic lenses about six millimeters in size, which are slid into the capsule behind the iris, usually as soon as the cataractous lens is removed. A stitch or two is needed to close the opening. With the less popular intracapsular method, an implant can still be used, but it must be placed in front of the iris. That is a more difficult procedure, with a greater chance of complications.

The preference for implants has had somewhat of a negative impact on phacoemulsification, a type of extracapsular surgery that its originators hailed as the next breakthrough in cataract removal. A titanium needle vibrating back and forth about 40,000 times a second breaks the cataract into tiny pieces, almost liquefying the lens with ultrasonic vibrations. The fragments are then sucked out through an incision that's several millimeters smaller than the one made for the extracapsular procedure. The bottom line is supposed to be a faster healing time.

A disadvantage may be that when the patient chooses an implant, that oh-so-small incision has to be widened to accommodate the larger synthetic lens.

The Need for Eyeglasses

Because the implant can't focus like the natural lens did, spectacles will probably be needed after surgery. "Despite our best efforts, there may be a small amount of astigmatism, or of nearsightedness or farsightedness, so we tell patients before surgery that they may need glasses in some instances," says Dr. Bogorad. "They usually don't mind, though, because they're willing to put up with glasses if it means getting their sight back." Adds Dr. Lubkin, "Contacts may be used in some cases, but they are more a nuisance for people in this age group."

Implants aren't for everyone with cataracts, however. The plastic lenses are usually restricted to people about 50 years of age or older. "The track record shows that implants are excellent for at least 30 years, but after that, we don't know what changes, if any, occur," says Dr. Bogorad. "With younger people, we usually recommend contacts."

There are other factors that could rule you out as an implant recipient. If you have problems with the initial cataract-removal surgery, you may have to settle for glasses or contacts. Cornea or iris problems or a history of retinal disease may also disqualify you from consideration for implants.

While most people walk away from the procedures with at least 20/40 vision, which is considered safe for driving in most states, many realize perfect 20/20 vision, adds Dr. Shulman.

In the months and years following extracapsular surgery, there's a 20 to 30 percent chance that the back of the capsule will cloud over. This is when a laser may be used. "People mistakenly think that cataracts can be burned out with a laser, but it's not possible. The laser is a secondary tool used months or years after the initial surgery. A few bursts are used to open a hole in the clouded capsule, which results in an immediate vision improvement," says Dr. Shulman. Where a laser isn't available, the clouded part of the capsule is surgically opened.

After surgery and follow-up visits to an ophthalmologist, there's something you should know. Sunlight and some forms of artificial light contain ultraviolet (UV) radiation, which may damage the retina, the sensitive inner lining of the eye that holds nerve fibers used for seeing. Your natural eye lens protected the retina from this radiation, but it was removed during surgery.

Shielding Your Eyes

What you need is some form of radiation shield between your eyes and the sun, and this is where eyewear is crucial. "Ordinary glass or plastic eyeglasses and sunglasses don't provide the needed UV protection," says Donald Pitts, O.D., Ph.D., a researcher at the University of Houston's College of Optometry. "There are special clear or tinted lenses that must be worn."

The UV-filtering glasses can be specially made by an optician or may be purchased off the rack. (Some of the newer implants have built-in UV protection, but the older models don't. Contact lenses offer no protection, either.)

"If you buy eyeglasses in a store, make sure they are designated Z80.3," which means they have met federal standards for UV protection, says Dr. Pitts. "These glasses filter out 95 percent of harmful radiation."

Wearing these glasses when outdoors may also slow the formation of some cataracts. "It's not only a good idea, it's necessary, in my opinion," says Dr. Pitts. "You can protect yourself from a lot of damaging radiation by wearing the right glasses. But you shouldn't wait until you reach the age of 40. Young people in their twenties should wear UV-protecting eyeglasses to prevent early damage."

Dr. Bogorad adds that buying inferior sunglasses without adequate UV protection is not a good idea. "Because sunglasses darken the area in front of the eyes, the pupils dilate, so even more radiation than normal could get into the eyes. It's not wise for any eyes, regardless of whether you've had cataract surgery, to be exposed to excess ultraviolet radiation."

Countering Cataracts with Nutrition

Although the research is still in the embryonic stages, nutrition may become another means of preventing cataracts. U.S. Department of Agriculture scientists at Tufts University Human Nutrition Research Center on Aging in Massachusetts have found preliminary evidence that some vitamins and minerals may guard the eye lens from the damaging action of sunlight and oxygen.

After working with laboratory animals, the researchers report that dietary vitamin C seems to concentrate in some eye lenses, preventing sun and oxygen from oxidizing proteins that might otherwise be involved in cataract formation. These workers are also trying to determine the role of other antioxidants and cofactors such as vitamin E, manganese, zinc and magnesium.

Pain Relievers Help Keep Eyes Clear of Cataracts

When you take aspirin for a headache, you probably don't have visions of it saving your sight. But it may have just that effect, according to new research by doctors in England.

Researchers at the University of Oxford compared the medical histories of 300 cataract patients with those of over 600 people without cataracts. Their surprising finding? A possible protective effect of long-term use of common pain relievers. The risk of cataracts is more than halved in people who take aspirin, acetaminophen, ibuprofen and related compounds, they found. The research also confirmed previous studies in which diabetes, glaucoma and steroid medications were found to be risk factors for developing cataracts. And the anti-angina drug nifedipine was found to carry increased risk.

The doctors aren't sure why pain relievers reduce the risk of cataracts, but they suspect it has something to do with the drugs' effect on blood sugar. "Aspirinlike analgesics lower fasting blood glucose levels . . . .They improve glucose tolerance . . . and the insulin response to glucose," they say, adding "that high levels of glucose predispose toward cataract is demonstrated . . . by the high risk of cataract in diabetic patients."

The researchers are starting a new study to determine just how much of these drugs it takes to have a protective effect. Another study of the effect of low doses of aspirin is also under way. But the research probably won't stop there. "If aspirinlike analgesics can protect against cataract by a modest lowering of plasma glucose, what other damaging effects of glucose do they diminish?" the researchers ask (*Lancet*).

If all goes well, dietary recommendations that could extend the life of the eye lens may be forthcoming within the next few years.

Considering the strides made so far, perhaps it's conceivable that someday medical science will come up with a way to predict whose sight will be affected by cataracts. Presently, there's no way to tell. If you have diabetes or an enzyme deficiency, if you have been taking cortisone for a long time, if you suffered an eye injury or have a family history of cataracts, your chances are slightly higher than those of the general population. But in most cases, you just have to wait and see.

CHAPTER 5

Modern Medicine against Stroke

Science is improving the odds of deterring, detecting and overcoming this physical cataclysm.

Because of research advances, more stroke victims than ever are surviving. Over the past 20 years, stroke deaths have dropped 40 percent.

And many survivors—even those with severe handicaps—are learning to walk again and talk again, getting ready to lead independent lives.

Medical research has also done much to prevent strokes from occurring. Scientists now know major risk factors that can lead to a stroke and have developed ways to treat many of them. Public health campaigns have taught the public that good health habits can help prevent stroke. So can knowing the warning signs of stroke and getting prompt medical care.

The Making of a Stroke

The occurrence of a major stroke is dramatic. A seemingly healthy person is felled by an invisible foe. Describing her near-fatal stroke, dancer and choreographer Agnes de Mille remembers: "I stood in the auditorium of the Hunter College Playhouse in New York City giving last-minute instructions to my dance company. Suddenly I discovered that half of my body was dead."

In reality, a stroke is not a bolt from the blue. It is instead often the symptom of an already existing condition that affects the flow of blood to the brain.

Unlike other organs of the body, the brain cannot store energy. It depends on a continuous supply of fresh blood pumped to it by the heart. A hefty 25 percent of the blood that the heart pumps goes to the brain.

If blood flow to a section of the brain stops for any reason, brain cells in the area lose their source of energy and begin to die. The result is a stroke.

In the most common form of stroke, the flow of blood is disturbed as an artery serving the brain gradually becomes clogged. Eventually the artery may become closed entirely by the formation of a clot.

The mass that forms within the artery is called a *thrombus,* the Greek word for "clot" or "lump." A stroke produced when blood supply to the brain is blocked because of such a clot is called a thrombotic stroke.

A brain artery can also be blocked or plugged by a clot that has formed elsewhere in the body, usually in the heart or the arteries of the neck, and is carried in the body's bloodstream to the brain. This kind of traveling clot is called an *embolus* (a Greek word for "plug").

Another word physicians use when discussing different types of stroke is *infarct.* When a clot blocks a blood vessel, the nerve cells served by that vessel are starved of blood-borne fuel and oxygen and within minutes begin to sicken and die. The dead cells, other debris and the clot itself accumulate into a mass of tissue called an infarct. Infarct strokes account for two-thirds of all cases.

Another 12 percent of all strokes occur when a blood vessel ruptures and blood pours into the brain. Uncontrolled bleeding of this sort is called hemorrhage.

Hemorrhagic strokes are usually more severe than infarct strokes. Not only is the blood supply to the brain cells lost, but the brain tissue itself is damaged by the escaped blood. Agnes de Mille's stroke resulted from a hemorrhage deep in the center of the left side of her brain—an often fatal event.

Certain rare blood diseases, inherited disorders and birth defects can also cause stroke. Some people, for example, are born with a weak section in the wall of an artery in the brain. The constant pressure of blood being pumped through the artery may cause the weak section to form a bulge called an *aneurysm.* The bulge may become so filled with blood that it bursts. Blood then floods into the brain and the victim suffers a stroke.

However it happens, a stroke of any type is a medical emergency. It demands immediate expert care.

Stroke survivors experience a variety of symptoms, depending upon what part of the brain is damaged. Some patients may be unable to speak or understand speech. The medical name for this problem is aphasia.

Other people are permanently paralyzed by stroke. But even severely affected people make partial recoveries. Some stroke survivors recover completely. How the brain recovers and what physicians—and patients and family members—can do to encourage recovery are among the leading questions that are challenging research neuroscientists today.

The Warning Signs

The number one goal of stroke research is to prevent stroke. Fortunately, nature has given science some help. Strokes are often preceded by warning signs that can be identified by a person who knows what to look for. The four most common warning signs of a stroke are:

- Transient numbness, tingling or weakness in an arm or leg or on one side of the face.
- Temporary blindness in one or both eyes.
- Temporary difficulty with speech.
- Loss of strength in a limb.

These are the symptoms of the transient ischemic attack—the so-called TIA—which, if left untreated, can lead to a major stroke.

Other danger signals are unusual or unexplainable headache, dizziness, drowsiness, nausea or vomiting. Abrupt personality changes and impaired judgment or forgetfulness will also warn the alert observer of possible impending stroke.

Such warning signs may be brief. The symptoms of light-headedness, feeling ill, numbness or memory loss may last only a few seconds, but it is wise not to ignore them even if they go away. The fact that the symptoms have disappeared does not mean that there is no medical problem.

Neither does the fact that TIA symptoms may occur infrequently. "One TIA is as menacing as many," one stroke specialist has warned.

It is best to see a physician immediately and be sure.

Getting a Diagnosis

The physician's job is to determine whether the symptoms you describe mean that you have had a stroke or may have one soon. Often this evaluation can be done in the physician's office. But in an emergency you might go directly to a hospital, where you would report your symptoms and medical history to emergency room physicians. That information plus routine tests and a neurological examination might be enough for them to make a tentative diagnosis of a stroke.

But sometimes the patient is unconscious. Sometimes, too, people have symptoms that look like stroke as a result of reactions to drugs or following an epileptic seizure. A delayed reaction to a head injury and certain kinds of brain tumor can also cause strokelike symptoms.

Emergency room physicians will discuss these possibilities with neurologists. They will conduct further tests to rule out conditions other than stroke that might be causing the symptoms. The tests will also help them distinguish between a thrombotic and a hemorrhagic stroke (a "plug" or a "leak," as some doctors call them), an important step since treatment for each type of stroke differs.

There are several tests that are commonly used to establish the diagnosis of stroke.

CT scan. Many neurologists believe that computerized tomographic (CT) scanning has revolutionized the diagnosis of stroke. This painless technique uses a computer to construct black-and-white pictures of the brain, obtained from multiple x-rays beamed through the head. An area of dead brain tissue as small as half an inch across can be seen and readily distinguished from an area that is bleeding. CT scans can be performed within minutes after a person arrives at a hospital. Physicians can order more scans later to gauge the effectiveness of treatment and to evaluate the course of healing. The CT scan is harmless for patients and gives the physician important information to use in providing the best possible care.

Arteriography. Arteriography produces extremely clear and detailed pictures of the main trunks and fine interconnected branches of the brain's treelike arteries. These pictures are called arteriograms.

The technique requires opening an artery and threading a flexible tube through the artery toward the neck. Then a liquid is injected into the artery. This liquid will show up on x-ray films made as blood circulates in the brain.

If you are to have an arteriogram, you will be advised that there is a small risk of injury, infection or allergic reaction to the injected material. You should also be told that thousands of arteriograms are performed safely every year. Physicians generally believe that for most patients the benefits of arteriography are greater than the risk.

DIVA. A safe, relatively new technique of x-raying brain arteries is called digital intravenous angiography

(DIVA). In this technique, the physician injects contrast liquid directly into a vein. A computer codes the x-ray images in numbers, with each number reflecting a different intensity of lightness or darkness. The computer then sharpens or enhances the difference between images taken before and after the contrast liquid is injected.

The pictures that result are not as detailed as arteriograms, but the technique is convenient, fast and safe. It is especially useful for patients too ill to undergo standard arteriography. It can also be used to screen stroke patients to determine who needs an arteriogram.

Ultrasonography. Many physicians use ultrasound equipment to look for defects in arteries of the neck, for these arteries are major suppliers of blood to the brain.

In this painless technique, a device placed on the patient's neck beams sound waves through the skin. A computer records and analyzes the echoes that bounce back as the sound waves are absorbed and reflected by the tissue.

Treating Stroke with Drugs

As soon as the physician knows that a patient has had a stroke and can determine what kind, treatment can begin. The physician's main concern is that the brain should suffer no further loss in circulation. Blood flow to the brain must be maintained and steps taken to prevent further damage.

In the case of an infarct stroke, strong drugs like heparin and warfarin may be prescribed for short-term use to prevent blood clots from becoming larger. These drugs are called anticoagulants.

Aspirin may also be used by certain stroke patients. But patients who have a history of ulcers should ask their physician whether using aspirin is wise. Usually, aspirin is of help to stroke-prone patients, but in people with stomach trouble, aspirin can sometimes cause bleeding.

A stroke caused by a ruptured aneurysm—the "hemorrhagic" stroke—may require treatment with drugs that preserve the blood clots that form at the rupture site. These clots are needed to plug the injury. Drugs that reduce brain swelling or control high blood pressure also may be prescribed.

Research has shown that many stroke patients become depressed—some only mildly; others to the point of despair. "Everything is so slow," said one stroke patient. "I've never been in a place that I couldn't get out of. What scares me the most is the fear of being a cripple."

This "poststroke depression" is most likely to occur between six months and two years after the stroke. About half of the severely depressed patients experience such symptoms as anxiety, loss of energy, weight and appetite, and sleep disturbances. This depression is partially due to the brain's reaction to the stroke and is partially a psychological reaction. Scientists are now testing a variety of drugs for this problem.

Making Your Way Back

Once the stroke patient is out of danger and vital signs are stable, rehabilitation should begin. Sometimes stroke survivors lose the benefits of rehabilitative treatment because they don't realize they should have it, they don't know where to find it or they don't continue treatment long enough to see lasting improvement.

Rehabilitation is a team effort. It involves the coordinated activities of physicians, physical and occupational therapists, social workers, speech and language specialists and other experts and counselors who work with the family as well as the patient.

After only a week in bed, muscles start to deteriorate. Physical therapy helps the patient strengthen muscles, improve balance and coordination and relearn the movements necessary for sitting, standing and walking. When needed, a variety of mechanical aids—walkers, crutches, canes and lightweight splints or braces—provide additional support.

Some patients experience the bizarre symptoms of "hemispheric neglect." As a result of one side (or hemisphere) of their brain being damaged, they ignore half of their body and the corresponding half of their visual world. Sometimes they deny that the neglected half even exists. Asked to put on a robe, the patient may insert an arm into only one sleeve. Asked to draw a human figure or the face of a clock, the patient may draw only half a body or a clock with the numbers crowded in on one side.

Hemispheric neglect can usually be overcome with training, but it may take the concerted effort of all members of the rehabilitation team and the family.

Speech and language therapists work with stroke patients who have sustained damage in the speech centers of the brain. Occupational therapists concentrate on improving eye/hand coordination and strengthening skills needed in writing, using tools and preparing food. Occupational therapy rooms are usually equipped with model kitchens and a variety of tools and gadgets designed for use by disabled people.

Rehabilitation experts are finding more and more evidence that a key element in patient rehabilitation is family support and encouragement. Research scientists in comprehensive stroke centers established by the National Institute of Neurological and Communicative Disorders and Stroke have found that training local community members to make home visits to stroke patients and counseling family members in rehabilitation methods seem to have paid off in better survival rates. Also, stroke patients in the research programs scored higher than expected in such areas as "activities of daily living."

Surgery for Stroke

Sometimes surgery can help stroke victims—surgery like the extracranial/intracranial bypass. When a clogged artery is located within the brain, a surgeon usually cannot operate to remove the obstruction. But sometimes a surgeon can perform the bypass to reroute blood past the clogged area.

In this operation, a healthy scalp artery at the top of the head (*extracranial* means "outside the skull") is passed through a hole in the skull to the brain inside (intracranial).

There it is joined to the clogged brain artery just beyond the obstruction. Blood then flows from the heart through the scalp artery and into the brain artery, bypassing the clogged area in much the same way that motorists use a detour to bypass a traffic jam.

Scientists do not suggest that this bypass is the answer for every stroke patient. You should talk with your doctor to see if this is an option for you.

Preventing a First—or Second—Stroke

In stroke, there is nothing so important as prevention. Survivors of a first stroke do not want to be among the 20 to 25 percent who suffer second or third strokes. Family members may wonder if they, too, will have a stroke and want to know what to do to prevent it. Fortunately, research scientists have identified several risk factors that can alert you before a stroke occurs.

High blood pressure (hypertension). A common and important risk factor for stroke is high blood pressure, which strains the heart and the walls of the arteries. High blood pressure is found in 70 percent of hemorrhagic stroke cases. Fortunately, early detection of hypertension and a growing number of medications are helping to bring this risk factor under control.

However, many stroke victims do not have high blood pressure. The absence of hypertension is no assurance that one is immune to stroke.

Atherosclerosis. If a physician says you have atherosclerosis, that means lumps of fatty substances have built up on the inside of your arteries, making them thick, rough and less flexible.

Atherosclerosis may begin in childhood. Examinations of soldiers in their twenties and thirties who were killed in Korea and Vietnam confirmed that in many, fatty deposits called plaques had already developed around the heart and in the large artery arising from the heart. In time, plaques occur in more distant arteries, bunching up especially at points where the arteries branch. Such a major junction occurs in the carotid arteries in the neck. That is why so much attention focuses on these arteries as sources of clots that can plug brain arteries.

Many neurological scientists are studying how atherosclerosis affects blood circulation within the brain. They have learned, for example, that when stroke is due to hypertensive atherosclerosis, about one-fifth of the survivors are left with varying degrees of dementia. Dementia is the neurological disorder associated with a loss of mental skills.

Heart disease. Common heart ailments such as coronary artery disease and valve defects often result in clots that may break loose and be carried by the blood into the brain.

Diabetes. Diabetes is commonly considered a disease affecting only the body's ability to use sugar. But it is also associated with destructive changes in blood vessels throughout the body. Diabetic patients are therefore at risk for developing a stroke. Equally serious, if their blood sugar is high at the time of the stroke, brain damage is usually more severe and extensive than when blood sugar is normal or low.

Obesity. Excess weight burdens the heart and blood vessels and increases the risk of heart disease, high blood pressure and diabetes. If the overweight person's diet is rich in salty foods, fats and cholesterol, so much the worse, for these ingredients can contribute to high blood pressure and atherosclerosis.

Lack of exercise. A sedentary life may not in itself cause a stroke but often is a companion to obesity. Even moderate amounts of exercise may strengthen the heart and improve circulation. Exercise may even help dissolve atherosclerotic plaques.

Other risks. Other factors that have been implicated in stroke are continued high levels of stress, hereditary disorders that lead to the accumulation of fat or cholesterol in blood, sickle cell anemia and other blood disorders. Use of birth control pills, particularly for a long time and in those who smoke, has also been associated with an increased tendency to form blood clots.

New Hope from New Research

On the horizon, researchers see new possibilities in the prevention and treatment of stroke.

PET. Positron emission tomography (PET) is a new technique for producing pictures of the brain. But these brain images are different from the pictures obtained through x-rays. X-rays show how the brain looks—its anatomy. PET, on the other hand, shows how the brain works—its chemical activity, or metabolism.

PET scanning relies on the need of active brain cells to burn glucose as fuel. Scientists can attach a harmless radioactive tag to glucose. This tagged glucose is injected into a vein and the PET scanner shows where the glucose goes once it reaches the brain.

The most active brain cells use the most fuel, so they will absorb the greatest amounts of glucose. Without causing the patient any pain, detectors outside the patient's head can identify sites where large amounts of glucose are being used. The detector does this by recording the amount of radioactivity that the cells at these sites give off.

A computer then translates these measurements into a color-coded image of the brain: The most active cells appear as light or bright areas, and less active or diseased tissue appears darker.

Aspirin studies. Several research studies have suggested that small daily doses of aspirin can protect against stroke by lessening the severity or number of transient ischemic attacks.

Normally a tear or other injury in a blood vessel wall serves as a signal that attracts certain small particles, called blood platelets, to the injury site. The platelets stick to the vessel wall, sealing the leak or covering the injury. They then manufacture chemical messengers that summon still more platelets to the scene, where they clump together.

Aspirin interferes with an enzyme the platelets use to manufacture these messengers. Platelets are then less likely to clump, and a clot is less likely to form and obstruct blood flow to the brain.

Atherosclerotic stroke patients appear to have especially "sticky" platelets, ready to clump together at the slightest provocation. That provocation is provided by the fatty plaques that line arterial walls: The plaques dig into the wall, causing injuries that call the platelets into action.

Aspirin has been shown to be effective in preventing thrombotic stroke. But experts have yet to decide what amount of aspirin would be most effective, or even if aspirin is the ideal drug to prevent stroke.

Aspirin studies have reawakened interest in a chemical called prostacyclin. This chemical is manufactured in muscle cells in the artery wall. Like aspirin, prostacyclin inhibits the clumping of platelets. The substance is being studied as a possible treatment for stroke.

Fish-oil diets. The cod-liver oil you may have had to swallow as a child may turn out to have unexpected benefits in stroke prevention for adults. Observers have long noted that people whose diet is rich in fish, like the Eskimo, seldom suffer heart attacks or strokes. Investigators have turned their attention to a particular ingredient in fish, eicosapentaenoic acid. They think this acid may somehow protect against atherosclerosis.

Endorphin studies. The brain may react to injury by releasing certain natural substances called endorphins. The endorphins are chemicals important in the control of pain. Some experiments suggest that they may also lower blood pressure. If so, brain tissue damaged by a stroke—an injury that promotes the production of endorphins—might get less blood and suffer even greater damage. Following that lead, some investigators are experimenting with agents that block the action of endorphins. In this way they hope to improve blood circulation in the stroke patient's brain.

CHAPTER 6
Medical Progress Report: Parkinson's Disease

There's encouraging news about early detection and possible prevention of this crippling motion disorder.

Diane Ruby's whole body shook after she was involved in a fender-bender several years ago. It was nerves, her doctor told her. But her right hand never really stopped trembling, and when her right leg started to drag two years later, she knew something was terribly wrong. Her friends convinced her to see a new doctor. His diagnosis, Parkinson's disease, came as a mixed blessing. Diane knew she wasn't going to die, at least not soon. But she also knew her life would never return to normal. Slowly, she would become more and more handicapped.

Parkinson's is a disease of the central nervous system that hinders the body's ability to move. Its victims—1 person in 100 over age 60 gets it—may experience a gradual and subtle onset of symptoms, such as a little shakiness or general slowing down, and may dismiss them as part of growing old. Gradually, they may find it hard to write or to button clothes. They may find it difficult to begin motions like walking or standing up. Their face may take on a fixed expression. Their hands may make movements as if they were rolling a pill between their fingers and thumb. It's often the hand tremors that get them to a doctor.

Younger people, like Diane Ruby, may find that their symptoms first appear after major stress—childbirth, surgery or an accident. Ten to 20 percent of Parkinson's victims have their first symptoms before age 50.

The disease is caused by damage to cells in a small part of the deep middle brain known as the substantia nigra. These cells produce a brain chemical called dopamine, which helps many other cells within the brain send messages involving muscle movement. As the cells die, dopamine levels drop. Other parts of the brain can't function properly, and so more and more symptoms appear.

Toxins May Play a Role

Exactly why these brain cells die isn't known. Many researchers believe it's a combination of aging, genetic tendencies and environmental triggers.

With aging, some of these cells are lost faster and earlier than usual. But aging by itself is not enough to explain accelerated cell loss.

Most studies of twins have shown no genetic tendency toward Parkinson's. But recent research by Andre Barbeau, M.D., of the Clinical Research Institute of Montreal, suggests that some people may be particularly prone to the disease. These people lack certain liver enzymes that help neutralize toxins taken in by the body.

Dr. Barbeau believes environmental toxins like insect and weed killers may be linked to the cell damage that leads to Parkinson's disease. He has observed in Canada that more cases of Parkinson's are found in commercial agricultural areas with high pesticide use. He thinks the chemicals may cause "clinically silent damage" to the brain. When that damage is followed by the normal cell loss of aging, symptoms may appear.

Intrigued by these studies, U.S. researchers plan to do similar work with liver enzymes to see if the findings hold, says Franz Hefti, Ph.D., associate professor of neurology and pharmacology at the University of Miami and director of research for the National Parkinson Foundation.

"It's a brand-new area that needs to be explored," Dr. Hefti says. "It gives us hope that in the future we might be able to identify people at risk for Parkinson's disease with a simple test."

Another test, a brain x-ray called positron emission tomography (PET), can detect low dopamine levels that result from the death of cells in the substantia nigra before the first symptoms of Parkinson's appear. "In the future, this test, which is just a research tool now, might be used regularly to screen people at risk for Parkinson's," says J. William Langston, M.D., director of Parkinson's disease research and clinical programs at the Santa Clara Valley Medical Center and the Institute for Medical Research, both in San Jose, California.

There will also be more studies of the connection between Parkinson's disease and environmental toxins, says William Weiner, M.D., professor of neurology and director of the Center for Movement Disorders at the University of Miami.

"We already know of some toxins," he says. People exposed to heavy concentrations of manganese in mills or mines, or those who have been knocked out by carbon monoxide, are more likely to develop a neurological disease like Parkinson's.

One finding that makes a chemical connection more of a possibility is that in the last few years, several people have developed all the symptoms of Parkinson's after taking a form of synthetic heroin called MPTP. This narcotic drug contains a compound that is structurally similar to some industrial chemicals and to the herbicide paraquat, which is sometimes sprayed on marijuana plants. These inadvertent human guinea pigs are providing researchers with a unique chance to study the cause, effect and treatment of Parkinson's.

Drugs Make Life Easier

Unfortunately, right now there is no proven way to prevent or cure Parkinson's disease, even when it is detected early. Its symptoms, though, can be controlled, sometimes for the remainder of a normal lifetime, with drugs.

"Once you get over the multitude of brand names, there

are basically four different compounds," says Dr. Hefti. The main drug is levodopa, or L-dopa. (A common brand name is Sinemet.) L-dopa is used by the body to make dopamine. It helps the remaining substantia nigra cells beef up their production of dopamine by providing them with plenty of building materials.

"L-dopa is an amino acid found in small amounts in strange tropical fruits or plants that hardly anyone ever eats," Dr. Hefti says. People with Parkinson's can't rely on food sources for the amounts they need.

Unfortunately, L-dopa becomes ineffective in 50 percent of patients within five to ten years after they start treatment. For that reason, many doctors prescribe it only when symptoms have begun to interfere with daily life. Then they give only enough to keep symptoms tolerable. Sometimes they'll have patients take the drug more often, without increasing the dosage. The first timed-release L-dopa formula, Sinemet CR, has been undergoing testing.

Often, doctors add to the L-dopa a second group of drugs, known as dopamine agonists. The most common brand name is Parlodel (chemical name, bromocriptine). These drugs are chemically similar to dopamine and act as a substitute for it. By themselves, though, they don't work as well as L-dopa.

A third group of drugs is known as anticholinergics. These drugs don't have a direct effect on dopamine production. Instead, they help to balance another brain chemical, acetylcholine, which is involved in the brain systems that control movement. With Parkinson's disease, there tends to be excessive activity of nerve cells releasing acetylcholine. Blocking that effect, at least in part, with anticholinergics helps to alleviate symptoms such as tremor and inability to start movements. Some doctors start out with anticholinergics, then move on to L-dopa.

A fourth compound, amantadine (Symmetrel), seems to act like anticholinergics, although no one is sure exactly how it works. Originally used as an antiviral drug, it was found to reduce tremor in Parkinson's patients, although it doesn't work as well as the other drugs.

Almost every L-dopa drug on the market contains a compound called carbidopa. By itself, carbidopa does nothing for the symptoms of Parkinson's disease. But added to L-dopa, it prevents much of the drug from being destroyed in the gut before it has a chance to reach the brain. It also decreases nausea and vomiting.

Reports come out now and then on some other drug or nutrient that seems to help Parkinson's symptoms. L-methionine, an amino acid, added to L-dopa, seemed to improve movement, muscle strength, mood and sleep in a study by researchers at the University of Alabama. Nicotine provides a very temporary (only minutes long) lifting of symptoms. Some antidepressants, and sometimes tryptophan, also seem to help. Some doctors also prescribe tyrosine, which is believed to have a mild effect like L-dopa, or lecithin, which they think might improve mobility and mental performance in certain Parkinson's patients.

But don't look for miracles among these other substances, Dr. Hefti warns. "None of them works as well as those currently being used."

Symptoms versus Side Effects

The symptoms of Parkinson's are actually fairly straightforward and easy to control with drugs, Dr. Weiner says. It's trying to minimize drug side effects that requires a fine, and increasingly difficult, balancing act over a lifetime.

The most common side effect of long-term L-dopa use is dyskinesia—involuntary dancelike movements and facial expressions. Psychiatric problems, such as vivid nightmares and hallucinations, may also occur. Depression is common. "Keeping dosages low and switching drugs helps to alleviate side effects," Dr. Weiner says. Taking a "drug holiday"—stopping drugs altogether for a few weeks—is no longer often recommended, he says. "It creates a lot of stress for the patient with only very temporary improvement."

None of the drugs currently marketed in the United

States for Parkinson's slows the disease's progress. Some researchers, in fact, worry that the drugs actually accelerate cell death.

"There's no doubt that people who take these drugs do live longer," says Dr. Langston. "L-dopa is so effective in reversing the symptoms that the disease may not shorten your normal life span. But the fact is, you may also be paying a price. The price is worth it, but sooner or later you'll probably have side effects from the medicine."

How? "One theory is that the oxidation of dopamine in the brain might somehow contribute to the death of nigral neurons," Dr. Langston says. "Oxidation happens in normal metabolism, but it's speeded up when the few cells remaining in the substantia nigra are forced to beef up production to meet demand. The process of oxidation creates destructive particles called free radicals. These particles may eventually destroy brain cells."

That's the reason researchers hope to study vitamin E, an antioxidant, for the role it might play in slowing the progress of Parkinson's disease. "Theoretically, it might work," Dr. Langston says. "Studies will show whether or not it really does work."

Researchers also plan to take a close look at a very interesting drug called deprenyl. This drug, a monoamine oxidase B inhibitor, is not yet available by prescription in the United States. But it has been used for about ten years in Europe to treat the symptoms of Parkinson's disease. It seems to be moderately effective against symptoms when given with L-dopa.

But what really interests U.S. researchers are two findings about deprenyl.

First, when European researchers reviewed their data, they were surprised to find that Parkinson's disease appeared to be progressing more slowly in people taking deprenyl. "These researchers concluded that monoamine oxidase inhibitors were actually slowing the progress of nigra-cell death," Dr. Langston says. "This study was retrospective and is suggestive—but not proof."

Second, when U.S. researchers tried giving deprenyl to

animals that were then exposed to MPTP, the animals developed none of the symptoms of Parkinson's.

"We found that MPTP in itself is not toxic to brain cells," Dr. Langston says. "It is not until MPTP is metabolized in the body and converted to another form that it kills brain cells. Deprenyl prevents MPTP from becoming toxic. It dramatically prevents brain-cell death in animals given MPTP."

Dr. Langston has begun a study to look at the role of deprenyl in Parkinson's disease. His work may become the pilot for a national study organized by researchers at Columbia University in New York City and at the University of Rochester. That study will look at both deprenyl and vitamin E as possible protectors against toxins and brain-cell death in Parkinson's disease.

If there's any message Parkinson's researchers want to get across, it's one of hope and excitement.

"A few years ago, you would never have heard anyone talking about the theoretical possibility of preventing Parkinson's, at least not seriously," Dr. Langston says. "Now we can detect it with the PET scan before symptoms appear. And if either one of these trials, with deprenyl or vitamin E, shows that there is a way to prevent further cell death, you could actually intervene and prevent symptoms from ever appearing at all. In years to come, the pieces might fit together very nicely."

Dr. Langston is just waiting for that day. So is Diane Ruby.

For more information, write to the National Parkinson Foundation, 1501 NW Ninth Avenue, Bob Hope Road, Miami, FL 33136, or call their hotline at (800) 327-4545. The foundation is affiliated with the University of Miami School of Medicine. Or contact the United Parkinson Foundation at 360 West Superior Street, Chicago, IL 60610, or call (312) 664-2344.

CHAPTER 7

Today's War on Irritable Bowel Syndrome

Doctors now say that most people who have this chronic digestive disease can alleviate their symptoms with careful attention to diet, stress management and exercise.

Sandy had stomach trouble for as long as she could remember. Minor bouts of nausea, diarrhea, constipation and cramps had come and gone for most of her 25 years. But it never lasted long enough and was never severe enough for her to seek medical help.

But suddenly that changed. For the last couple of months the alternating diarrhea and constipation were almost nonstop, and the abdominal cramps were becoming more and more painful. The frequent trips to the bathroom and the constant discomfort were the last thing she needed, because her new job was terribly demanding.

Sandy's family doctor could find nothing wrong with her. And a visit to a gastroenterologist, a doctor who specializes in digestive diseases, turned up the same result. Other than her symptoms, there was nothing physically awry. Sandy had a very typical case of irritable bowel syndrome.

Irritable bowel syndrome, also known as spastic colon, is the most common of all the digestive diseases. It's more common than ulcers, ulcerative colitis, ileitis, hepatitis, cirrhosis of the liver, gallbladder disease, inflammation of the pancreas and hiatal hernia. It affects an estimated 20 to 25 million people in the United States. Yet the cause remains unknown.

Even though doctors don't know *why* it's happening, they do know *what* is happening. "Individuals with irritable bowel syndrome have a supersensitive stomach, small intestine and large intestine," says Arnold G. Levy, M.D., associate clinical professor of medicine at George Washington University Medical Center in Washington, D.C., and a member of the presidential National Digestive Disease Advisory Board. "They have an exaggerated response to what they eat and drink, and to stress." Irritable bowel syndrome is known as a functional disorder because there is no physical disease of tissues but rather an abnormality in the function of the digestive system.

Disorderly Conduct

Normally, the muscles from the esophagus to the end of the large intestine contract rhythmically in a process known as peristalsis, which moves food through the digestive tract in an orderly fashion. But in people with irritable bowel syndrome, the contractions lose their pattern. They're no longer synchronized or coordinated. And they may become more intense. So there is no normal progression of food downstream. These people also secrete excess stomach acid.

The excess acid causes a gnawing sensation in the stomach, a feeling of constant hunger, heartburn, indigestion and nausea, especially early in the morning. The abnormal contraction or cramping of the intestinal tract is experienced as abdominal pain.

If the cramps are intermittent and irregular, the person will probably have diarrhea. If the cramps are constant and continuous, the result is constipation. "Typically, people with irritable bowel syndrome have alternating constipation and diarrhea," explains Dr. Levy, who is also vice-president for education for the American Digestive Disease Society. "They'll feel well for a day or two, then feel terrible and have diarrhea for a couple of days, then things will settle down and they'll be constipated for a couple of days. The cycle will repeat and they'll never feel totally well."

In fact, contractions can be so bad that the person becomes a prisoner of the bathroom. "Many people with irritable bowel syndrome have to be very careful where they go," Dr. Levy says. "They have to know exactly where the bathroom is in a shopping center or supermarket because they don't know when they're going to have an attack. You can imagine how distressing it can be if your whole life revolves around where the bathroom is."

Bellyachers

Most doctors agree that irritable bowel acts up in response to stress and the ingestion of foods that produce intestinal gas. "There are no definitive studies proving exactly what goes haywire," says David M. Taylor, M.D., a gastroenterologist in Atlanta and clinical assistant professor of gastroenterology and medicine at Emory University and at the Medical College of Georgia. "But the symptoms do get worse during periods of stress. It's the most common trigger."

Gas-producing foods also trigger episodes because they distend areas of the intestinal tract. "This doesn't bother most of us," Dr. Levy points out, "but in people with irritable bowel syndrome it causes a reflex contraction, and they start to feel miserable very quickly."

Other foods can also cause problems for people with irritable bowel syndrome. Some doctors think that it is totally idiosyncratic—different foods cause intestinal spasms in different people—and that you can't make generalizations. But other doctors disagree. "Caffeine and anything fried, fatty, greasy or oily will make things worse for almost everybody with irritable bowel syndrome," Dr. Levy maintains. "Garlic will also cause problems. As a general rule of thumb, though, if an individual identifies a specific food that he or she can't handle, it's best to stay away from it."

Although certain things aggravate the condition, the root cause remains elusive. "We can clearly say that stress does not cause this condition," says Dr. Levy. "It just makes it worse. The same is true of diet."

We do know that irritable bowel syndrome is more common in women (about two-thirds of the people with the disease are women), that it usually begins between the ages of 20 and 40, and that it is not at all dangerous. "The condition is serious only in the fact that it is disturbing to the patient," says Marvin M. Schuster, M.D., director of the Gastrointestinal Division at Francis Scott Key Medical Center and professor of medicine and psychiatry at Johns Hopkins University School of Medicine in Baltimore. "It can be socially and professionally disruptive, and it can prevent people from doing things they want to do. But it doesn't lead to shortened life, it doesn't lead to cancer, and it doesn't lead to ulcerative colitis. People with irritable bowel syndrome don't lose weight (unless they're also depressed) or become dehydrated or malnourished. They have lots of distress, lots of discomfort, but they're otherwise quite healthy."

Luckily, there are a number of things that can ease that discomfort. Doctors don't agree on all of them, but they do seem to agree on one of them: fiber. "A high-fiber diet is absolutely the cornerstone of treatment," says Dr. Taylor.

Dr. Levy agrees. "The thing that works best to control spasms is to increase the amount of bulk in the intestinal tract. That's done by increasing the amount of fiber in the diet," he says. "It makes a big difference for almost everybody with irritable bowel syndrome.

"The usual content of the American diet is about 10 grams of fiber daily. By some recommendations it ought to be about 40 grams. But the addition of even 5 to 10 grams of fiber is sometimes all that is needed to make all the difference in the world in settling things down. The increased bulk decreases the intensity and frequency of the contractions and promotes smoother passage through the entire intestine.

"The fiber can be provided by whole wheat bread, bran muffins, bran flakes or other high-fiber cereals, miller's bran or fiber supplements," recommends Dr. Levy. "Psyllium-seed powders such as Metamucil, Hydrocil and Fiberall can be mixed into juice or water and consumed once or twice a day. Each provides about 3½ to 5 grams of fiber per teaspoon. Another source is fiber cookies, such as Fibermed or Fiberall. Each cookie contains about 5 grams of fiber. There's even a fiber candy on the market. Each candy provides about 3.4 grams of fiber. It's important to let people know that they have several good alternatives, because some individuals may have trouble increasing the fiber in their diet."

That may just be the case with someone who has irritable bowel syndrome, because avoiding gas-producing foods such as broccoli, cabbage, brussels sprouts, cauliflower, beans, onions and lentils can mean passing up some good sources of fiber. It also means passing up some good sources of vitamins and minerals. That's why the American Digestive Disease Society's dietary plan cautions irritable bowel syndrome patients to use appropriate supplements if their diet is extremely limited.

"If the addition of fiber and the avoidance of caffeine and fatty, gassy and other irritating foods don't manage the condition, then antispasmodic medications may be used," says Dr. Levy. "They work to decrease the spasms going through the intestinal tract. Patients can use them until things quiet down, then go off the drug and only use it when needed. But the best thing is control and prevention."

A Positive Outlook

Control and prevention don't end with diet, though. Because irritable bowel syndrome is triggered by stress, finding ways to reduce stress is important. That can start right at the doctor's office. "It's important to develop a feeling of mutual cooperation with the patient," says Dr. Schuster. "That's best done by having an interest in the person and his problem and in helping him to overcome it.

"It's important to dispel any misconceptions and explain that irritable bowel syndrome is a chronic condition that's rarely cured. You can keep it in check, but occasionally it breaks through. If the patient understands that, he or she won't worry that it's developing into cancer or something else whenever it flares up. Worrying only makes it worse."

Dr. Schuster also tries to teach patients not to focus on irritable bowel syndrome all day long any more than they'd focus on any other physical complaint. "It's not good for them to tell everybody on the corner what their complaints are," he says. "Their spouses and families can help, too. I ask them not to reinforce sick behavior but instead to reinforce healthy behavior. And I try to get the patients to push themselves to their maximum performance.

"To alleviate stress, I help patients identify the stressors—the factors in their lives that are producing stress," says Dr. Schuster. "Then they can try to remove them in the most logical fashion. If they're in the wrong job, for instance, it may be possible to leave it. Or if they find that they can't leave, they may just need to learn some coping techniques to manage the situation."

"Lifestyle changes are very important to handling stress," adds Dr. Taylor, who is coauthor of *Gut Reactions—How to Handle Stress and Your Stomach*. "In my opinion, working it out physically is the best thing. Running, bicycling, aerobic exercising and other sports are most important.

"When people with irritable bowel syndrome gain control of their lives, they get a lot better. Not necessarily 100 percent better—the problem seems to wax and wane. But they can get a lot better by understanding, by insight, by controlling their own lives."

Therapies That Help

Psychotherapy may help some people gain that insight and control. In a Swedish study, over 100 patients with irritable bowel syndrome were put into two groups. Both groups received the same medical treatment, but patients in one of the groups also received ten hour-long psychotherapy sessions that focused on means of coping with stress and emotional problems. After three months the patients in the group receiving psychotherapy had significantly greater improvement in their symptoms. What's more, they had improved even further after a year had gone by, while the patients who received only medical treatment got a little bit worse.

"The combination of medical treatment with psychotherapy improves outcome, not only in the short term but also in the long run," say the researchers (*Lancet*).

In a study done in England, doctors compared the effectiveness of psychotherapy and hypnosis in treating patients who were not helped by the usual medical measures. In that study, reported in the journal *Lancet*, the patients receiving hypnotherapy aimed at general relaxation and control of intestinal activity showed dramatic improvement in all symptoms. And their improvement was significantly greater than the improvement showed by patients receiving psychotherapy.

"In individuals in whom stress is the key factor aggravating their condition, stress management and relaxation training are an absolutely key part to their therapy," says Dr. Levy. "Counseling, psychotherapy and biofeedback to reduce stress can all be very helpful. I have sent several patients whose conditions were unmanageable in any other way for hypnosis. Some have done very nicely and some have not responded well. I look at it as another one of several ways of managing stress."

"Anxiety and depression are more common in people with irritable bowel syndrome than in others," Dr. Schuster says. "We don't know whether that predisposes someone to having the disease, but it certainly makes it worse. For that reason, very low-dose antidepressant medication is helpful in some patients, because of both its antidepressant effect and its calming effect on the gut. But most patients with irritable bowel syndrome don't need to see a psychiatrist. Only those who would need to see a psychiatrist anyway—if they don't have irritable bowel syndrome—should see one."

Accurate Diagnosis a Must

According to Dr. Taylor, irritable bowel syndrome is diagnosed when a patient has abdominal cramps and changes in bowel habits, such as diarrhea or constipation, and sometimes nausea, without any signs of serious disease, like fever, weight loss or bleeding. The symptoms have usually been present for over six months with no change, and all tests have turned out normal.

"If the intestines are inflamed, the blood tests will show it," Dr. Schuster explains. "And the person may have a fever. And since there are no structural changes associated with irritable bowel syndrome, any bleeding means it's something else (unless the bleeding is caused by hemorrhoids or fissures)."

According to Dr. Levy, irritable bowel syndrome used to be a diagnosis of exclusion. "The doctor would do every test and every x-ray under the sun. If all of the tests and x-rays were negative, they'd call it irritable bowel syndrome. It's clearly recognized now that that's not necessary."

"X-rays are generally not done so much nowadays," confirms Dr. Schuster. "Instead, a fiberoptic colonoscopy [inspection of the lining of the colon, using a flexible tube with a light at the end] can be done to rule out organic, physical causes.

"Another basic thing to rule out is lactose intolerance, which can mimic irritable bowel syndrome in every fashion," he says. "If the symptoms disappear after two weeks on a lactose-free diet, it's purely a lactose problem."

"Lactose, or milk sugar, is a double sugar that must be split in two in order to be absorbed," Dr. Levy explains. "It's broken down in the intestinal tract by an enzyme called lactase. If there's not enough lactase, the lactose passes undigested all the way through 25 feet of small intestine into the colon. There, bacteria ferment it to produce lactic acid, a colon irritant, and carbon dioxide gas."

Because both lactose intolerance and irritable bowel syndrome are very common, a person might very well have both conditions.

"Forty percent of patients with irritable bowel syndrome have some degree of lactose intolerance, which aggravates their condition," Dr. Schuster says.

"Everyone with irritable bowel syndrome should try a lactose-free diet for two weeks to see if it makes a differ-

ence," he continues. Lactose is present in dairy products and in foods prepared with dairy products, such as bread, pastry, cakes and cookies. And Dr. Levy mentions that it is also used in some vitamin tablets as a filler.

If you would like more information about irritable bowel syndrome and helpful dietary measures, write to the American Digestive Disease Society, 7720 Wisconsin Avenue, Bethesda, MD 20814, and enclose $1 for postage and handling.

CHAPTER 8

Countering the Ancient Ailment Called Gout

Kings and sultans suffered from the painful joint disease, but nowadays there are ways you can avoid it.

Open any history book, flip to the chapter on kings and what do you see? Usually puffy cheeks, a neck the size of a tree trunk and stately robes wrapped around what looks like a barrel with arms. Once upon a time, gluttony reigned supreme, and skinny kings were as common as dragons.

The feasting that went along with the job carried a price, however, and more than a few monarchs suffered the excruciating pain—often in the big toe—that seemed to follow a royal repast. All the king's men never could quite deduce that the food and wine and his majesty's girth were aggravating a recurring disease of the joints, what we now call gout.

Today gout is a more democratic disease, crossing social strata and causing pain and discomfort for nearly two million Americans, mostly middle-aged men, from all walks of life. It is still one of the most misunderstood arthritic ailments, often misdiagnosed and confused with one of the other 100-odd types of arthritis. Yet, enough is now known about the centuries-old ailment to help many modern men avoid or at least reduce the number of attacks. Scientists have found, for instance, that controllable factors such as diet, obesity, alcohol, stress and even otherwise beneficial pharmaceuticals can cause gout episodes. The permanent crippling that once afflicted many can now be avoided.

But to understand gout is to understand a substance that a Swedish apothecary discovered in 1776 while doing research in the kitchen of his herb shop after hours. That substance is uric acid.

Acid and Needles

The body naturally manufactures purines, which are also found in some foods. Purines break down in the body and form uric acid in the blood, which in most people is carried to the kidneys for removal. When there's too much uric acid—a condition called hyperuricemia—it comes out of solution and forms microscopic, needlelike crystals in the joints. The crystals may also make their way to the kidneys, where they can form kidney stones or affect the organs' function by damaging tissue.

"It's like putting too much sugar in iced tea," says Jeffrey R. Lisse, M.D., a rheumatologist and assistant professor of medicine at the University of Texas Medical Branch, Galveston. "When there's a lot of sugar, the crystals don't dissolve and just fall to the bottom of the glass. In the case of uric acid, the excess crystals wind up in the joints."

Scientists suspect that any fluctuation of uric acid dislodges these crystals, somewhat like waves moving sand on a beach. The movement of these crystals causes what is more commonly known as a gout attack.

Some cases of gout are the result of an inborn metabolic defect that causes an overaccumulation of uric acid—either too much is produced or it's not excreted adequately. It's suspected that most gout victims' problems with uric acid are inherited and that if you shake the family tree, gouty ancestors will fall out. While children of a parent with gout may not develop the disease, their chances are greater than those of the rest of the population.

Gout may also develop as a complication of some other disorder, such as diabetes, psoriasis or leukemia.

"Most gout victims are similar to diabetics. They unknowingly have the right conditions for the disease but don't realize it until all the circumstances are right. Then some factor causes a fluctuation of uric acid levels and triggers an attack," says Dr. Lisse.

In the case of gout, that trigger can come in a variety of forms. Excess weight is often associated with increased uric acid levels. Also, overweight people often take hypertension (high blood pressure) medication, which could trigger an attack.

"Drugs for treating hypertension, which are being used by more people these days, can also affect the kidneys' ability to function properly and cause a uric acid increase," says Armin Good, M.D., a rheumatologist and professor of medicine at the University of Michigan, Ann Arbor, and chief of the Arthritis Section at Ann Arbor Veterans Administration Hospital. "Alcohol has a well-documented effect and gets you both ways: It impairs excretion and also causes an overproduction of uric acid."

Any factor that puts stress on the body can cause a change in uric acid levels and loosen those painful urate crystals. "Dehydration, infections, even surgery can cause a flare-up of gout," says Dr. Lisse. Even a drug designed to lower uric acid levels during an attack can be administered too fast and cause a rapid change, thus triggering another painful episode. Strenuous exercise, a bodily injury, thiazide diuretics, emotional stress and fatigue can also affect uric acid levels.

When these fluctuations occur, the big toe is often a prime target but not the only sore point. The pain of gout can be felt in almost any joint, including the neck, ankle, instep, wrist, elbow, knee and fingers, to name a few. Once the crystals are in the joint, the body's white blood cells that normally fend off unwanted invaders attack and remove the crystals. More microcrystals are deposited, however, unless the uric acid levels remain under control and don't fluctuate.

The disease affects mostly middle-aged men and is considered rare in males 20 to 30 years of age. Women are usually safe until after menopause, when hormonal changes cause an increase in uric acid levels. Even so, the number of women afflicted is only a small percentage of the total number of gout cases.

So it should come as no surprise that lists of famous sufferers are usually devoid of women's names: Henry VIII, Michelangelo, Leonardo da Vinci, Alexander the Great, Martin Luther, Sir Isaac Newton, Benjamin Franklin and John Milton, whose vivid descriptions of hell in *Paradise Lost* are said to have been inspired by his suffering. The aches of such luminaries were attributed to a too-rich diet, but chances are the high-purine meals were probably only a contributor, not the cause.

Is It Really Gout?

It's difficult for the average aching person to tell whether their discomfort is gout, rheumatoid arthritis or another musculoskeletal disorder, since these conditions share similar symptoms. With gout, inflammation is accompanied by a throbbing pain that often begins at night. The joint becomes swollen and tender and the skin is hot, turning a shade of red or purple. "If it flares up and goes away in a few days, it may be gout," says Dr. Good. "If it persists, it could be another form of arthritis, although this isn't a definite rule of thumb."

Checking uric acid levels in the blood isn't always a good indicator, either. "Many a misdiagnosis has been made based on a blood test," says Dr. Lisse. "The test may show that a person has high levels of uric acid, so the doctor will start the patient on drug treatment. But it's possible to have high uric acid blood levels and never show any gout symptoms. So you have a person taking an expensive drug that has possible side effects, and they may not need it."

The best test for gout simply requires inserting a needle into the affected joint and drawing fluid that's examined under a microscope for the telltale crystals. "It's the simplest test in the world and prevents delay and needless suffering," says Dr. Good. "Any competent rheumatologist can do it, but more skill is required if the gout is in small joints, such as those below the ankle."

In most cases, the initial attack is usually mild, involving one joint and vanishing in a matter of days or a week. The next attack could be weeks, months or even years away for some people. For the unfortunate, the attacks are more frequent. If misdiagnosed and not treated as gout, more joints gradually are affected and the pain intensifies. Gout that goes untreated can lead to a buildup of uric acid crystals in the joints and the formation of rocklike chunks called tophi, which can eat away bone and cause irreversible damage.

Several drugs are commonly used to treat gout, the most popular being colchicine, probenecid and allopurinol. All can have unpleasant side effects. Once prescribed, probenecid and allopurinol must be taken continuously. "It's not something that should be addressed lightly, because you'll be taking a drug for life," adds Dr. Lisse.

Draining the Pool

If you've already experienced the painful throbbing and have thought of ordering an official Henry VIII gout stool for propping up swollen appendages, don't—it's not too late to improve the odds for the future. Says Dr. Good, "A person could reduce the size of their uric acid pool and possibly prevent or at least reduce the number of attacks. Granted, some people are genetically predisposed and will have gout regardless of what they do. But they are the minority. And for those people treatment is highly successful. The others could probably spare themselves some of the pain with a few lifestyle changes."

Besides watching your weight and eliminating alcohol,

limit the amount of purine-rich foods you eat. To avoid attacks, gout sufferers should stay away from the following foods, which have approximate purine contents that range from 150 to 1,000 milligrams per 3½-ounce serving: anchovies, asparagus, brains, consommé, gravies, heart, herring, kidney, liver, meat extracts, mincemeat, mushrooms, mussels, sardines and sweetbreads.

If you're prone to gout, you should also limit your intake of the following, which have purine contents of 50 to 150 milligrams per 3½-ounce serving: dried beans and peas, cauliflower, fish, lentils, meats, oatmeal, poultry, seafood, spinach, whole grain cereals and yeast.

The effects of purine-rich foods and alcohol were reinforced a few years ago when researchers at the University of Pittsburgh School of Medicine offered seven gout patients a banquet fit for medieval royalty. When dining without alcohol, the volunteers' uric acid levels increased slightly, but they jumped drastically when whiskey or wine accompanied the meal.

Be forewarned, however, against a weight-loss diet that radically reduces food intake. Research has shown that severely cutting back, and especially fasting, stresses the body and can increase uric acid levels.

Drinking more water, probably several more glasses a day, can help. The fluid dilutes the uric acid's harmful effects and also helps the kidneys excrete it. Plenty of fluids also help avoid kidney stones, which can form when uric acid crystals clump together.

Some gout sufferers claim to have found relief with cherries. Canned, fresh and frozen cherries—even cherry juice concentrate—have all helped some people, or so they say. The remedy was first described by a scientist named Ludwig Blau in the late 1940s. A gout victim himself, Blau one day was nibbling on a bowl of cherries and noticed his pain had disappeared. He found that the discomfort didn't return as long as he kept cherries on the menu.

For those gout victims with a sweet tooth and a penchant for folk remedies, Blau's fruit cure may sound appealing. For those who prefer more credible scientific data, there's enough for the medical community to conclude that painful gout attacks are preventable. With what we now know, perhaps the lists of famous and not-so-famous sufferers will see few, if any, future additions.

CHAPTER 9

Silencing the "Noise in Your Ears"

At last there's relief for the unwanted sounds in your ears known as tinnitus.

For years, the standard medical "treatment" for buzzing, ringing or roaring noises in your ears was no treatment at all. Your doctor would say you'd just have to learn to live with it.

For some, that might have been easier said than done. Unwanted ear noise, known as tinnitus, has been reported to reach volumes as high as 70 decibels. That's equivalent to having a vacuum cleaner in your head. It's no wonder that some sufferers who couldn't learn to live with it instead chose a quick exit.

Today, new and better diagnosis and treatment can help alleviate many of the symptoms of tinnitus.

Doctors divide tinnitus into two types. Objective tinnitus can be heard not only by the victim but also by another listener. Doctors sometimes use a stethoscope with two earpieces to listen to the noises in their patients' ears. Objective tinnitus can be a throbbing or rushing noise from a circulation problem near the middle ear or clicking from a muscle spasm in the throat or jaw.

Usually, though, only the victim hears the noise. This is known as subjective tinnitus because it's being generated by ear nerves that for one reason or another have decided to play their own tune. The noise may be temporary—

brought on by a loud noise, sinus congestion or a change in altitude. When it becomes a permanent fixture, though, it's more likely to have been caused by changes in the aging ear or long-term exposure to noise. Most people first notice a faint buzzing or roaring when they lie in a quiet room at night. It's likely to be accompanied by some hearing loss in the high-frequency range, which many people don't notice, at least initially.

Tinnitus and the Aging Ear

Degeneration in the aging ear is a leading cause of tinnitus. With it comes some hearing loss.

"As the ear ages, it becomes susceptible to cell damage," says Simon Parisier, M.D., chairman of the Department of Otolaryngology at Manhattan's Eye, Ear and Throat Hospital. The seashell-shaped inner ear, called the cochlea, is particularly prone to aging-related damage and hearing loss. The cells lining this organ can stiffen and die. Circulation problems may block off its blood supply. Diabetics are particularly prone to hearing loss, and Dr. Parisier believes they may suffer the same kind of circulatory damage to their inner ear as they do to their eyes, where broken capillaries leak blood into the retina.

"It's important to look at the inner ear as part of the total body," Dr. Parisier says. That means keeping diabetes and blood pressure under control, improving circulation by lowering blood-fat levels, losing weight if necessary and checking for proper thyroid function, glucose metabolism and general good nutrition. Dr. Parisier often works with a patient's family doctor or internist if he suspects the tinnitus or hearing problem requires an overall approach. It's important to eliminate the rare possibility of a tumor on the auditory nerve, which most often causes a symmetrical (one ear only) tinnitus or hearing loss.

Loud Noises Can Last Forever

Exposure to loud noises accelerates aging changes. The sound waves of noise are turned into fluid waves in the inner ear. These waves sweep over the hair cells lining the inner ear. The cells' delicate microscopic nerve endings send signals to the auditory nerves, which go to the brain. Prolonged noise exposure slowly tears away at hair cells. Sudden blasts create a "tidal wave" effect in the inner ear.

A loud firecracker, a peak in already loud music or the incoming ring on a cordless telephone can blow hair cells away permanently. The ringing you hear as a result of these noises is your ear nerves, literally reverberating from the stress. Don't think your ears have to hurt to be damaged by noise.

Experts recommend you wear earplugs when you're on a motorboat or snowmobile, around power equipment or shooting a gun. If you use stereo headphones, take it easy on the volume. If you get stuck next to a loud portable radio or wailing infant, use the two very good earplugs you always have around—your index fingers. If you already have tinnitus, wear earplugs around shrill air conditioners, blenders and vacuum cleaners. Cotton won't protect your ears. Wear protective headphones or moldable foam earplugs.

Think of temporary tinnitus from noise exposure as a warning to protect your ears. It means that if you continue to be exposed to that volume of noise, you can expect permanent hearing loss and tinnitus that may not go away.

Earwax, Viruses and Drugs

Tinnitus can sometimes be caused by other factors. Earwax that is completely blocking the ear canal is simple to treat, although not a particularly common cause, Dr. Parisier says. Viruses that usually produce only a temporary hearing loss can trigger tinnitus. Anemia, blows to the head, high blood pressure, allergies (especially those causing congestion) and migraine headaches have also been implicated.

Caffeine is a more common culprit than many tinnitus sufferers realize, hearing experts say. Eliminating coffee, tea, colas and cocoa is all some people have to do to keep their symptoms under control.

Aspirin can cause ringing, or even worse. One elderly woman who complained to her doctor that she had been hearing "When Irish Eyes Are Smiling" playing in her head for several weeks was found to be suffering from aspirin-induced musical hallucinations, a rare form of tinnitus. She had been taking 12 aspirins a day for arthritis. Cutting back to 6 tablets a day cured her problem, saved her sanity and allowed her once again to appreciate her favorite song.

Some aspirin-related compounds, like bismuth subsalicylate and magnesium salicylate, can also cause tinnitus in susceptible people.

Antibiotics in the aminoglycosides family (the "mycin" group) have been associated with tinnitus. In a few very susceptible people, they may be particularly hazardous because they can cause permanent hearing loss long before tinnitus appears, some experts say. Hearing screening tests are suggested for people who are taking these antibiotics.

Treating Noise with Noise

Most people with tinnitus can't expect a cure, but they can get help for their symptoms. In many cases, a hearing aid that corrects for the hearing loss in the high-frequency range helps people reduce or eliminate their awareness of the tinnitus by focusing their attention on outside sounds.

Combining a hearing aid with a device known as a tinnitus masker, or using a masker alone if there is no hearing loss, is another possible treatment. The masker produces a high-pitched hissing noise to cover up the tinnitus. Success rates for maskers vary tremendously, with estimates ranging from 5 to 70 percent. Audiologists who recommend and fit them say the trick to success is to make sure the patient is a good candidate for a masker and that he's matched to the masker that's best suited for his problem. In some cases, people find that a masker has a residual effect, eliminating their tinnitus for several hours even after they have turned the masker off. (The masker does not interfere with hearing since the volume can be controlled.)

Some people with mild tinnitus have found that soft music, "environment" tapes of waterfalls, surf or rainfall, even the gentle hiss between stations on an FM radio, help mask their tinnitus and let them relax, especially at night, says Steven Berman, Ph.D., an audiologist and assistant professor at the Medical College of Pennsylvania in Philadelphia.

"You are introducing a sound that is simply a little bit louder than the sound they have inside their head," Dr. Berman says. "The brain is only going to hear the louder sound, not both."

Tuning Out Altogether

Most tinnitus victims find that their symptoms get worse when they're feeling stressed or when they focus their attention on their problem. Those are reasons relaxation training has worked well with some sufferers. "It can help people unwind and learn to turn their attention from their ear noise to more pleasant things," Dr. Berman says.

Drugs having an effect on the central nervous system have been tried for tinnitus, but their performance has been mostly disappointing, according to Dr. Berman. Most doctors try to avoid using drugs for tinnitus.

Reassurance is still a factor in tinnitus, Dr. Parisier says. "After you have taken a patient's symptoms seriously and looked for all causes, you can often reassure him that his problem isn't going to hurt him or get worse. That may be enough to allow him to adapt and live with his symptoms."

And those who can't live with their symptoms—who are seriously disturbed by the noise in their head—need to know that they, too, can be helped.

CHAPTER 10

How to Read the Warning Signs on Your Skin

By Howard Donsky, M.D.

Understanding the outside indicators of inside disease can save your life. A dermatologist tells you what to look for.

Only a small percentage of the skin problems I see turn out to be signals of internal disease, but you can imagine my feelings when they are noticed on an unsuspecting person. Early investigation of such signs has saved many people's lives over the past 19 years of my dermatology practice. I hope this fact alerts you to the significance of danger signals on your skin. The earlier you notice something wrong, the faster you can get it investigated and treated, and the longer you may live.

Diabetes

Diabetes, a metabolic disease, causes these changes in the skin.

- Circular, cordlike, pinkish brown or flesh-colored thickening of the skin. This is known as granuloma annulare. It can be a single lesion or is sometimes found all over the body.

Dr. Howard Donsky is associate professor of medicine (dermatology) at the University of Toronto and staff dermatologist at Toronto General Hospital.

- Yellow, waxy plaques on the shins, with spiderlike blood vessels coursing like rivers through the waxy surface. This is known as necrobiosis lipoidica diabeticorum.
- Infections of the skin are more frequent in diabetics and, when they occur, they tend to be more inflamed and angrier than normal.
- Little yellow bumps appearing on any portion of the body, particularly on the eyelids and over the joints. They are caused by higher-than-normal cholesterol levels and are known as xanthomas.
- A yellow-orange skin tone due to elevated levels of carotene in the blood, particularly evident on the palms.
- Severe itching.
- Increased hair and pigmentation on the face near the temples. Irritation and inflammation of the skin at the corners of the mouth, called perlèche. A loss of skin pigmentation, called vitiligo.
- The appearance of ulcers on the feet is one of the most dangerous results of diabetes. Because the disease causes damage to the arteries that carry oxygenated blood to the tissues, the resulting lack of oxygen can cause tissue breakdown. The nerves in the feet lack nourishment and lose their sensitivity. Any hurt to the feet can then go unnoticed and ulcerate. Ulcers on the feet in diabetics are one of the most common reasons for amputation.

  If you are diabetic, be sure to follow these steps to prevent ulcers from appearing on your feet: Wear well-fitting leather shoes and thick cotton socks; use lots of talcum powder on your feet and inspect your feet frequently; be very careful about pedicures, making sure that your toenails are never cut too closely; and never go about in bare feet.
- Loss of hair on the lower legs and decreased pulse in the lower parts of the legs are also caused by vascular abnormalities.
- Although not common, there are two other skin problems that can happen in diabetics. Sometimes a lost ability to sweat (anhidrosis) can cause dry skin and an

inability to deal with extreme heat. Another condition that can occur is scleredema, in which there is swelling of the skin about the face, neck and upper trunk. Not all people with scleredema are unhappy about the condition; this plumped-out skin can give them a more youthful appearance.

Thyroid Malfunction

When a hyperactive thyroid gland condition, called hyperthyroidism, is present, there are a number of signals from the skin.

- Increased sweating.
- Increased or decreased pigmentation.
- Itchiness and swelling of the shins, sometimes accompanied by redness.
- Separation of the nails and clubbing, a thickening of the skin around and under the nails.
- Loss of hair, either in patches or over the entire scalp.

A decreased function of the thyroid gland, called hypothyroidism, can be signaled by the following:

- Dry and sometimes thickened skin over the entire body.
- A yellow-orange coloration in the skin, particularly in the palms.
- Little yellow bumps on the eyelids and joints, called xanthomas.

The hair and nail conditions that occur in hyperthyroidism can also occur in hypothyroidism, as can hair loss on the ends of the eyebrows.

Adrenal Disease

The following changes in the skin occur when the adrenal gland is hyperactive, a condition known as Cushing's syndrome.

- Puffiness of the eyelids.
- Increased hairiness and acne on the face, which becomes round and red (known as moon face).

- Skin that is thinned out, bruises easily, heals poorly and is easily infected.
- Increased deposits of fat on the trunk, while in contrast, the arms and legs are very thin.
- A fat deposit called a buffalo hump on the back of the neck.
- Purple stretch marks, or striae, on the trunk of the body.

A condition known as Addison's disease occurs when the adrenal glands are underactive. Signs of this disease are:

- Increased pigmentation of the skin and hair (the hair becomes darker). The deeper pigmentation is more noticeable on sun-exposed skin, areas of trauma such as the knees, elbows and scars, in the skin folds and in the creases of the palm. The vagina and mouth also show hyperpigmentation.
- There may be longitudinal bands of pigment down the nails.
- There is sometimes a tendency to decreased amounts of body hair, especially in the underarms.

Collagen Disease

There is a curious group of diseases called collagen, or connective-tissue, diseases, for which the causes are unknown. However, they seem to be autoimmune conditions, which means that an individual is allergic to some component of his or her own body.

Lupus erythematosus is the most common collagen disease and can affect almost any organ in the body, although the damaged organ most likely to endanger the person is the kidney. The most commonly affected organ is the skin, and it is skin changes that usually bring the patient to the doctor. It can start with a little red patch on the face that flares up in the sun and can continue on to deep, destructive scarring. It often takes the form of a butterfly-shaped pattern over the nose and cheeks. If you have lupus erythematosus, it's important to see your doctor. Although the skin eruption can seem relatively harmless, the rash can also be a harbinger of more serious systemic lupus erythematosus (SLE), which can damage any or all of the body organs or systems.

Gastrointestinal Disease

Several gastrointestinal conditions can be heralded by skin changes. The most important ones are listed below.

- If you develop an inflamed, ulcerated lesion in the mouth or one on the skin that is purplish in color with ragged edges, it could be an indication of ulcerative colitis. Red, tender nodules on the shins or inflammation of the veins, particularly on the legs, can also occur with this condition.
- Peutz-Jeghers syndrome, an uncommon condition in which frecklelike lesions appear on the lips and fingertips, is a sign of growths in the gastrointestinal tract. Fortunately, these growths are usually not malignant.
- Jaundice, dilated blood vessels on the skin (telangiectasia) and enlarged nipples in the male can be signs of cirrhosis of the liver.

Internal Malignancy

Metastases are clusters of malignant cells that spread to the skin from other areas of the body. This happens to 1 out of every 20 people who have an internal malignancy. The metastases reach the skin by three different routes: direct invasion of the tumor to the skin, as in breast cancer; via the lymphatic vessels; via the blood vessels.

The most frequent sites of origin for these metastases to the skin are, in order of frequency:

1. Skin
2. Breast
3. Stomach
4. Lung
5. Uterus
6. Kidney
7. Prostate

8. Ovary
9. Colon
10. Bladder
11. Thyroid
12. Thymus
13. Testicle

When cancer spreads to the skin, the area involved often indicates where the malignancy originated. For example, cancer on the scalp has generally spread from the breast, lung or genitourinary system; if it is on the chest, the cancer probably comes from the breast; if on the umbilicus, it comes from the gastrointestinal system; and if in the pubic region, from the genitourinary system.

Metastatic skin lesions are usually hard, nontender and nonulcerated nodules. They may be flesh-colored, pink, brown or occasionally even black. Less commonly, an ulceration of the skin or even a localized area of hair loss known as alopecia can be due to metastases. Occasionally there is an area of thick skin known as peau d'orange, because fibrotic thickening of the skin makes it resemble an orange peel. This type of metastasis is seen in breast cancer.

Inflammation of the skin of the breast, usually on the nipple, can be a sign of underlying breast cancer. Cancer must always be considered when only one nipple shows signs of dermatitis and does not respond to treatment with topical cortisone cream. In this situation, it is mandatory that a woman undergo a deep surgical biopsy to search for an underlying carcinoma of the breast. Her other breast should also be carefully examined, because there is an increased incidence of a second breast cancer in women who have had the condition in one breast.

Metastatic lesions on the skin often demonstrate the same characteristics on biopsy as the site they came from. For example, when examined under a microscope, the cells of a cancerous lesion in the skin will still resemble lung cells if they spread from that organ. The metastases may show up before the primary cancer has been discovered. In fact, in about half the cases where the original site of the cancer is in the lungs or kidneys, the metastases appear on the skin before the existence of the internal malignancy has been discovered.

Skin Inflammations

Although inflammations of the skin are a common occurrence, there are times when they signal internal diseases.

Certain types of itching can be danger signals, but because dry, itchy skin is a common complaint of the elderly in the winter months, a physician must judge whether the symptoms are unusual enough to warrant investigation.

Although its cause remains unknown, multiple sclerosis occasionally first begins with intermittent itching.

In a young or middle-aged individual, continuous itching on the feet and lower legs, which spreads to the lower half of the body or goes on to become a generalized itch involving the entire body, could be cause for concern. It might be a signal of Hodgkin's disease.

Itching that signals leukemia has a greater tendency to be generalized but is not as severe as in Hodgkin's. Bruises may develop due to bleeding into the skin, which may vary from small hemorrhages under the nails to large areas of the skin. They warrant investigation, especially if there has been no physical trauma to the involved areas. An anemic pallor noted at the same time usually points to leukemia.

When it occurs in adults over the age of 40, a collagen disease called dermatomyositis is a signal of internal malignancy in almost 50 percent of the cases. This association does not occur in children with the same condition. The skin changes seen in dermatomyositis include a violet-colored discoloration plus swelling of the eyelids, which resembles a sunburn. There are also transient red rashes, which can become more permanent, associated with dilated blood vessels, thinning of the skin and a mottled pattern of pigmentation.

Another type of pigmentation, in which the skin begins to look darker, can be a sign of extensive malignant melanoma or a tumor of the pituitary gland. Although rare, a generalized skin eruption with a distinctive pattern resembling wood grain, known as erythema annulare centrifugum, is almost surely a sign that an internal malignancy is present in the breast or lung.

Repeated episodes of flushing in the face, neck and upper chest, which last from 10 to 30 minutes and are accompanied by difficulty in breathing, abdominal cramps, explosive diarrhea and sometimes a severe drop in blood pressure, can alert a physician to a carcinoid tumor.

There are other skin conditions that can at times signal the presence of an internal malignancy. In most people, this will not prove to be the case, but I am listing them so that you will be aware of the possibility and go to a doctor for a diagnosis. It could save your life if you spot a danger signal early enough.

Other Danger Signs

Here are some other skin signals that should alert you to the possibility of problems elsewhere in the body.

- A thickening of the palms and soles in adults is occasionally a sign of Hodgkin's disease, leukemia or cancer of the esophagus or lung.
- A fish-scale type of skin (ichthyosis) beginning in an adult may be a sign of Hodgkin's disease.
- Extensive lanugo (soft and silky hair) on the face or body of an adult can be a rare sign of an internal malignancy, particularly in the lung or bladder.
- Brown, velvety discolorations in the body folds (usually in the underarms and groin) are an almost certain sign of internal malignancy if they occur in a thin adult. If this dirty-colored skin, which later becomes velvety and then rougher on the surface, appears in children or obese adults, it is usually benign.
- Clubbing of the fingers can be a sign of lung, heart or gastrointestinal disorders, including internal malignancy.

- A sudden shower or outcropping of rough brown spots, known as seborrheic keratoses, in an adult can be a sign of internal malignancy.
- Little (1/8 inch in diameter) hard pits that look like warts on the palms and soles can indicate internal malignancy due to the ingestion of arsenic years earlier. Localized types of skin tumors, which are also due to arsenic ingestion years before, can indicate internal malignancy as well.
- Poikiloderma is the name for skin changes consisting of a mixture of a mottled type of increased and decreased pigmentation along with dilated blood vessels and atrophy. It can occur in people who have been exposed to excessive amounts of x-ray irradiation. Another example of this kind of skin change can be seen in farmers or sailors who have been exposed to the sun for many years. The skin pattern may be benign or may be associated with various lymphomas or Hodgkin's disease. It can be present for many years before the underlying malignancy is discovered.
- There is a rare condition of the skin marked by large furrowed folds on the face, especially the forehead and eyebrows, caused by a thickening of the skin and bone. It can be associated with clubbing of the fingers and thickening of the palms. When this condition is seen in men over the age of 40, cancer of the lung is frequently present.
- Small blue, purple or brown nodules may be due to lymphoma-type skin malignancies. These are sometimes the first sign of acquired immune deficiency syndrome (AIDS). This contagious condition can be fatal and is now occurring in both the heterosexual and homosexual communities. The virus responsible is spread by contact with an infected person's body fluids.

CHAPTER 11
How to Subdue a Herpes Attack

New medical knowledge makes it possible to control this sexually transmitted disease.

Love may languish, but herpes is forever.

That—at least for now—is the evil truth about genital herpes, one of the shrewdest and most widely traveled viruses in the world. Researchers say a bona fide cure for the "love bug" is not even in sight.

But the good news is that the infection can be controlled. There are ways to make those agonizing flare-ups mind their manners. And there are ways to avoid passing the virus on to your partner without sacrificing your sex life altogether.

You may have heard about some things people have tried that doctors say *don't* work very well, including the amino acid lysine, sometimes used to treat cold sores, ointments whose active ingredient is zinc (like calamine lotion), lithium, BHT and meditation.

"Most of the holistic remedies—vitamins, diet, stress reduction and the like—help some people some of the time," says Marcus Conant, M.D., a leading herpes researcher at the University of California, San Francisco, School of Medicine.

But there's one thing that helps almost everyone, almost all the time: the prescription drug acyclovir (sold as Zovirax). "Acyclovir is the first scientifically proven, predictable way to control herpes," Dr. Conant says. "Taken as directed, under a physician's supervision, acyclovir is very effective and remarkably free from side effects."

The introduction of acyclovir ointment in 1982 offered

the first hope that the blisters, itching and pain of a herpes flare-up could at least be controlled, if not cured. From a medical standpoint, the development of a drug that controls a virus is a major breakthrough, as significant as the discovery of antibiotics, Dr. Conant says. Until now, he explains, viruses have been untouchable because they conceal themselves so well inside the body's cells. In effect, viruses are breaking-and-entering artists of the first order, breaking and entering the cell, then commandeering the equipment the cell uses to duplicate itself. Instead of turning out healthy new cells, the burglarized cell begins turning out new viruses. It's very difficult to develop a drug that will kill a virus without also killing the otherwise healthy cell. And although acyclovir *doesn't* actually kill the herpes virus, it's the first drug ever developed to prevent a virus from replicating.

Acyclovir is not a cure, but it's a drug that "manages" the disease, much as diabetes and hypertension are managed by medication. It comes in three forms (all available only by prescription): ointment, tablets and an intravenous solution that is used for people who have severe cases of herpes coupled with a weak immune system. The ointment, which was introduced first, is applied during initial outbreaks directly to the sores, with gratifyingly dramatic results. It speeds up healing and reduces the pain of the sores. But because it is applied only topically, the cream can't reach the virus cells lurking in the body, so it doesn't prevent recurrences.

The oral form of acyclovir has almost made that no-relapse dream come true for herpes sufferers. Taken regularly, the tablets make herpes flare-ups less frequent for most people and milder if they do occur. In a year-long study, nearly half of a group of Dr. Conant's patients who were given acyclovir had no recurrences at all.

The drug appears to be safe to take for a long period—a year, for instance—although no one knows for sure if there could be any unwelcome consequences of taking it for a lifetime. Fears that going off the drug might trigger severe attacks also seem to be unfounded, Dr. Conant says.

Curbing Contagion

Many people with herpes say the fear of infecting their sexual partner is the worst part of the disease. Until very recently, doctors assumed that the only time a herpes sufferer was contagious was during an actual attack or just before it. But a team of National Institutes of Health (NIH) physicians has described a case of herpes transmitted from an infected man to a previously healthy woman—despite the fact that he showed no visible signs of being infectious (*New England Journal of Medicine*). The researchers' depressing conclusion: You *can* pass herpes along even between flare-ups.

But Dr. Conant offers some reassurance here. For one thing, he says, regular acyclovir use probably reduces infectiousness (the man in the NIH case was taking it only intermittently). And only people with very active infections—with eruptions every month to six weeks—are likely to be infectious in this dormant phase. For another, he says, there are several simple things you can do to ensure that you don't pass the accursed bug along.

Using a condom lathered up with spermicide is one of the best and simplest ways to protect your partner. Spermicidal jellies that contain nonoxynol-9 (Orthocreme, Delfen, Conceptrol and others) are very effective at killing the herpes virus on contact, says Dr. Conant. "By using a condom lubricated with spermicide, you can reduce your risk of transmitting (or receiving) the virus." There is no scientific proof that you can completely prevent transmission this way, but both Dr. Conant and Robert Hatcher, M.D., of the Emory University School of Medicine, believe that this method affords enough protection to be worth the trouble. Dr. Hatcher cautions, though, that a condom only protects against the virus coming from sores on the penis itself in men, and on the cervix and vagina, not the external genitals, of women.

In fact, anything that kills the herpes virus on contact on the skin surface should help prevent transmission, says Dr. Conant. Even everyday organic solvents like alcohol or Campho-phenique would do the job, he notes. Then there is Zilactin, a nonprescription cold sore preparation sold in drugstores, which has become popular with herpes patients in California. The San Luis Obispo County Health Agency has handed it out in its sexually transmitted disease clinics for the past two years. Now the manufacturer hopes to distribute Zilactin nationally once the U.S. Food and Drug Administration approves it as a treatment for genital herpes. These topical remedies speed healing and relieve pain, but since they aren't antivirals, they won't prevent recurrences.

Another new topical over-the-counter drug that should be available in your local drugstore is an ointment called ImmuVir. Unlike the other preparations, ImmuVir contains an antiviral drug called InterVir. In tests involving over 150 patients, Charles B. Goldberg, M.D., of the Oregon Health Sciences University, found evidence that InterVir not only kills the herpes virus but may also strengthen the body's immune response to later attacks. While that is still only speculation, there is no doubt that InterVir relieves symptoms very quickly (in an hour or less, in most cases). It shortens the duration of an outbreak by about 2½ days and may also reduce the chance of infecting another person.

Cure Is a Long Time Coming

If the good news about herpes is that it can be controlled, the bad news is that a cure is a long way off. "There won't be a cure for herpes for at least 20 years," says Dr. Conant. "Antiviral research is still in its infancy. What we need in the meantime is a vaccine, and I'm not too hopeful about that, either."

He blames lack of progress toward a herpes vaccine on our lawsuit-happy times. "Every major drug company has been sued at least once. It will cost $30 million to develop a vaccine, and no one wants to risk losing that kind of time, money and work in a product-liability suit. A vaccine would be good for everyone: It would protect healthy people from getting herpes and relieve herpes sufferers of the fear of transmitting the disease. But until our society accepts that no drug can be entirely risk free for everyone, pharmaceutical companies are going to be reluctant to invest in research like that."

The story of herpes is pretty long on such depressing comments. But there's one bit of good news that may ultimately save you. After more than a decade of treating millions of people with herpes, doctors have noticed that very often the flare-ups become less severe and less frequent as time goes by. The virus seems to mellow with age. And though you'll never be entirely free of it (unless a cure is found), as the years go by, your herpes infection will be increasingly less likely to ruin your day.

CHAPTER 12
Stopping the Hurt of Headaches

Now doctors know more than ever about diagnosing, treating and preventing this common pain.

An estimated 40 million Americans experience chronic headaches. For at least half of these people, the problem is severe and sometimes disabling. It can also be costly: Headache sufferers make over 8 million visits a year to doctors' offices.

Fortunately, most victims of serious headaches can fight back. Medical science now knows more and can do more to ease the agony.

Why Does It Hurt?

What hurts when you have a headache? The bones of the skull and tissues of the brain itself never hurt because they lack pain-sensitive nerve fibers. Several areas of the head, however, can hurt, including a network of nerves that extends over the scalp and certain nerves in the face, mouth and throat. Also sensitive to pain, because they contain delicate nerve fibers, are the muscles of the head and blood vessels found along the surface and at the base of the brain.

The ends of these pain-sensitive nerves, called nociceptors, can be stimulated by stress, muscular tension, dilated blood vessels and other triggers of headache. Once stimulated, a nociceptor sends a message up the length of the nerve fiber to the nerve cells in the brain, signaling that a part of the body hurts. The message is determined by the location of the nociceptor. A person who suddenly realizes "My toe hurts," is responding to nociceptors in the foot that have been stimulated by the stubbing of a toe.

A number of chemicals help transmit pain-related information to the brain. Some of these chemicals are natural painkilling proteins called *endorphins,* a Greek word for "the morphine within." One theory suggests that people who suffer from severe headache and other types of chronic pain have lower levels of endorphins than people who are generally pain free.

When You Should See a Physician

Not all headaches require medical attention. Some result from missed meals or occasional muscle tension and are easily remedied. But some types of headache are signals of more serious disorders such as head injury and call for prompt medical care. These include:

- Sudden severe headache.
- Headache associated with convulsion.
- Headache accompanied by confusion or loss of consciousness.
- Headache following a blow on the head.
- Headache associated with pain in the eye or ear.
- Persistent headache in a person who was previously headache free.

- Recurring headache in children.
- Headache associated with fever.
- Headache that interferes with normal life.

A headache sufferer usually seeks help from a family practitioner. If the problem is not relieved by standard treatments, the patient may then be referred to a specialist—perhaps an internist or neurologist. Additional referrals may be made to psychologists.

Diagnosis: What the Physician Looks For

Diagnosing a headache is like playing "20 Questions." Experts agree that a detailed question-and-answer session with a patient can often produce enough information for a diagnosis. Many types of headaches have clear-cut symptoms that fall into an easily recognizable pattern.

Patients may be asked: How often do you have headaches? Where is the pain? How long do the headaches last? When did you first develop headaches? The patient's sleep habits and family and work situations may also be probed.

Most physicians will also obtain a full medical history from the patient, inquiring about past head trauma or surgery and about the use of medications. A blood test may be ordered to screen for thyroid disease, anemia or infections that might cause a headache. X-rays may be taken to rule out the possibility of a brain tumor or blood clot.

A test called an electroencephalogram (EEG) may be given to measure brain activity. EEGs can indicate a malfunction in the brain, but they cannot usually pinpoint a problem that might be causing a headache.

A physician may suggest that a patient with unusual headaches undergo a computerized tomographic (CT) scan. The CT scan produces images of the brain that show variations in the density of different types of tissue. The scan enables the physician to distinguish, for example, between a bleeding blood vessel in the brain and a brain tumor. The CT scan is an important diagnostic tool in cases of headache associated with brain lesions or other serious disease. Experts generally agree, however, that this sophisticated and expensive technology is not required to diagnose simple or periodic headache.

An eye exam is usually performed to check for weakness in the eye muscle or unequal pupil size. Both of these symptoms are evidence of an aneurysm—an abnormal ballooning of a blood vessel. A physician who suspects that a headache patient has an aneurysm may also order an angiogram. In this test, a special fluid that can be seen on an x-ray is injected into the patient and carried in the bloodstream to the brain to reveal any abnormalities in the blood vessels there.

Thermography, an experimental technique for diagnosing headache, promises to become a useful clinical tool. In thermography, an infrared camera converts skin temperature into a color picture, or thermogram, with different degrees of heat appearing as different colors. Skin temperature is affected primarily by blood flow. Research scientists have found that thermograms of headache patients show strikingly different heat patterns from those of people who never or rarely get headaches.

A physician analyzes the results of all these diagnostic tests along with a patient's medical history in order to arrive at a diagnosis. Headaches are diagnosed as vascular, muscle contraction, traction or inflammatory.

Vascular headaches—a group that includes the well-known migraine—are so named because they are thought to involve abnormal function of the brain's blood vessels or vascular system. Muscle-contraction headaches appear to involve the tightening or tensing of facial and neck muscles. Traction and inflammatory headaches are symptoms of other disorders, ranging from stroke to sinus infection. Some people have more than one type of headache.

Some Facts about Migraine Headaches

The most common type of vascular headache is migraine. Migraine headaches are usually characterized by severe pain on one or both sides of the head, an upset stomach and, at times, disturbed vision.

Basketball star Kareem Abdul-Jabbar remembers experiencing his first migraine at age 14. The pain was unlike the discomfort of his previous mild headaches.

"When I got this one, I thought, 'This is a headache'," he says. "The pain was intense and I felt nausea and a great sensitivity to light. All I could think about was when it would stop. I sat in a dark room for an hour, and it passed."

Symptoms of migraine. Abdul-Jabbar's sensitivity to light is a standard symptom of the two most prevalent types of migraine-caused headache, classic and common.

The major difference between the two types is the appearance of neurological symptoms 10 to 30 minutes before a classic migraine attack. These symptoms are called an aura. The person may see flashing lights or zigzag lines or may temporarily lose vision. Other classic symptoms include speech difficulty, weakness of an arm or leg, tingling of the face or hands and confusion.

The pain of a classic migraine headache is described as intense, throbbing or pounding and is felt in the forehead, temple, ear or jaw or around the eye. Classic migraine starts on one side of the head but may eventually spread to the other side. An attack lasts one to two pain-wracked days.

The common migraine—a term that reflects the disorder's greater occurrence in the general population—is not preceded by an aura. But some people experience a variety of vague symptoms beforehand, including mental fuzziness, mood changes, fatigue and unusual retention of fluids. During the headache phase of a common migraine, a person may have diarrhea and increased urination, as well as nausea and vomiting. Common migraine pain can last three or four days.

Both classic and common migraine can strike as often as several times a week or as rarely as once every few years. Both types can occur at any time. Some people, however, experience migraines at predictable times—near the days of menstruation or every Saturday morning after a stressful week of work.

The migraine process. Research scientists are unclear about the precise cause of migraine headaches. There seems to be general agreement, however, that a key element is changes in blood flow in the brain. People who get migraine headaches appear to have blood vessels that overreact to various triggers.

Scientists have devised one theory of migraine that explains these changes and also certain biochemical changes that may be involved in the headache process. According to this theory, the nervous system responds to a trigger such as stress by creating a spasm in the nerve-rich arteries at the base of the brain. The spasm closes down or constricts several arteries supplying blood to the brain, including the scalp artery and the carotids, or neck arteries.

As these arteries constrict, the flow of blood to the brain is reduced. At the same time, blood-clotting particles called platelets clump together—a process that is believed to release a chemical called serotonin. Serotonin acts as a powerful constrictor of arteries, further reducing the blood supply to the brain.

Reduced blood flow decreases the brain's supply of oxygen. Symptoms signaling a headache, such as distorted vision or speech, may then result, similar to symptoms of stroke.

Reacting to the reduced oxygen supply, certain arteries within the brain open wider to meet the brain's energy needs. This widening, or dilation, spreads, finally affecting the neck and scalp arteries. The dilation of these arteries triggers the release of pain-producing substances called prostaglandins from various tissues and blood cells. Chemicals that cause inflammation and swelling and substances that increase sensitivity to pain are also released. The circulation of these chemicals and the dilation of the scalp arteries stimulate the pain-sensitive nociceptors. The result, according to this theory, is a throbbing pain in the head.

Women and migraine. Although during childhood boys and girls seem to be equally affected by migraine, the condition is more common in adult women than in men.

Both sexes may develop migraine in infancy, but most often the disorder begins between the ages of 5 and 35.

The relationship between female hormones and migraine is still unclear. Women may have "menstrual migraine"—headaches around the time of their menstrual period—which may disappear during pregnancy. Other women develop migraine for the first time when they are pregnant. Some are first affected after menopause.

Migraine triggers. Fatigue, glaring or flickering lights, the weather and even certain foods can set off migraine. It may seem hard to believe that eating such seemingly harmless foods as yogurt, nuts and lima beans can result in a painful migraine headache. However, some scientists believe that these foods and several others contain chemical substances such as tyramine that constrict arteries—the first step of the migraine process. Other scientists believe that foods cause headaches by setting off an allergic reaction in susceptible people.

While a food-triggered migraine usually occurs soon after eating, other triggers may not cause immediate pain. Scientists report that people can develop migraine not only during a period of stress but also afterward, when their vascular systems are still reacting. The "Preacher Monday-Morning Headache" is named for those clergymen who get migraines a day after the stress of delivering a Sunday sermon. Migraines that wake people up in the middle of the night are also believed to result from a delayed reaction to stress.

Treating Migraine

During the Stone Age, pieces of a headache sufferer's skull were cut away with flint instruments to relieve pain. Another unpleasant remedy used in the British Isles around the ninth century involved drinking "the juice of elderseed, cow's brain and goat's dung, dissolved in vinegar." Fortunately, today's headache patients are spared such drastic measures.

Drug therapy, biofeedback training, stress reduction and

elimination of certain foods from the diet are the most common methods of preventing and controlling migraine and other vascular headaches. Regular exercise, such as swimming or vigorous walking, can also reduce the frequency and severity of migraine headaches.

During a migraine headache, temporary relief can sometimes be obtained by using cold packs or by pressing on the bulging artery found in front of the ear on the painful side of the head.

Drug therapy. There are two ways to approach the treatment of migraine headache with drugs: Prevent the attacks, or relieve symptoms after the headache occurs.

For infrequent migraine, drugs can be taken at the first sign of a headache in order to stop it or at least ease the pain. People who get occasional mild migraine may benefit by taking aspirin or acetaminophen at the start of an attack. Aspirin raises a person's tolerance to pain and also discourages clumping of blood platelets. Small amounts of caffeine may be useful if taken in the early stages of migraine. But for most migraine sufferers who get moderate to severe headaches, and for all patients with cluster headaches, stronger drugs may be necessary to control the pain.

One of the most commonly used drugs for the relief of classic and common migraine symptoms is ergotamine tartrate, a vasoconstrictor that helps counteract the painful dilation stage of the headache. For optimal benefit, the drug is taken during the early stages of an attack. If a migraine has been in progress for about an hour and has passed into the final throbbing stage, ergotamine tartrate will probably not help.

Because ergotamine tartrate can cause nausea and vomiting, it may be combined with antinausea drugs. Research scientists caution that ergotamine tartrate should not be taken in excess or by people who have angina pectoris, severe hypertension or vascular, liver or kidney disease.

Patients who are unable to take ergotamine tartrate may benefit from other drugs that constrict dilated blood vessels or help reduce blood vessel inflammation.

For headaches that occur three or more times a month, preventive treatment is usually recommended. Drugs used to prevent classic and common migraine include methysergide maleate, which counteracts blood vessel constriction, propranolol, which stops blood vessel dilation, and amitriptyline, an antidepressant.

In a study of propranolol, amitriptyline and biofeedback conducted by the Houston Headache Clinic, scientists found that migraine patients improved most on a combination of propranolol and biofeedback. Patients who had mixed migraine and muscle-contraction headaches received the greatest benefit from a combination of propranolol, amitriptyline and biofeedback.

Another study showed that propranolol may continue to prevent migraine headaches even after patients have stopped taking the drug. The scientists who conducted the study speculate that long-term therapy with propranolol may have a lasting effect on blood vessels, training them to react less than usual to the triggers of migraine.

Antidepressants called monoamine oxidase (MAO) inhibitors also prevent migraine. These drugs block an enzyme called monoamine oxidase, which normally helps nerve cells absorb the artery-constricting chemical serotonin.

MAO inhibitors can have potentially serious side effects—particularly if taken while ingesting foods or beverages that contain tyramine, a substance that closes down arteries.

Several new drugs for the prevention of migraine have been developed in recent years, including papaverine hydrochloride, which produces blood vessel dilation, and cyproheptadine, which counteracts serotonin.

All of these antimigraine drugs can have adverse side effects, but they are relatively safe when used carefully. To avoid long-term side effects of preventive medications, headache specialists advise patients to reduce the dosage of these drugs and then to stop taking them as soon as possible.

Biofeedback and relaxation training. Drug therapy for migraine is often combined with biofeedback and relaxation training. Biofeedback is a space-age word for a technique that can give people better control over such body function indicators as blood pressure, heart rate, temperature, muscle tension and brain waves. Thermal biofeedback allows a patient to consciously raise hand temperature. Some patients who are able to increase hand temperature can reduce the number and intensity of migraines. The mechanism of this hand-warming effect is being studied by research scientists.

"To succeed in biofeedback," says a headache specialist, "you must be able to concentrate and you must be motivated to get well."

In another type of biofeedback called electromyographic, or EMG, training, the patient learns to control muscle tension in the face, neck and shoulders.

Either kind of biofeedback may be combined with relaxation training, during which patients learn to relax the mind and body.

Biofeedback can be practiced at home with a portable monitor, but the ultimate goal of treatment is to wean the patient from the machine. The patient can then use biofeedback anywhere at the first sign of a headache.

The antimigraine diet. Scientists estimate that a small percentage of migraine sufferers will benefit from a treatment program focused solely on eliminating headache-provoking foods and beverages.

Other migraine patients may be helped by a diet to prevent low blood sugar. Low blood sugar, or hypoglycemia, can cause dilation of the blood vessels in the head. This condition can occur after a period without food—overnight, for example, or when a meal is skipped. People who wake up in the morning with a headache may be reacting to the low blood sugar caused by the lack of food overnight.

Treatment for headaches caused by low blood sugar consists of scheduling smaller, more frequent meals for the patient. A special diet designed to stabilize the body's sugar-regulating system is sometimes recommended.

For the same reason, many specialists also recommend that migraine patients avoid oversleeping on weekends. Sleeping late can change the body's normal blood sugar level and lead to a headache.

Beyond Migraine: Other Vascular Headaches

After migraine, the most common type of vascular headache is the toxic headache produced by fever. Pneumonia, measles, mumps and tonsillitis are among the diseases that can cause severe toxic vascular headaches. Toxic headaches can also result from the presence of foreign chemicals in the body. Other kinds of vascular headaches include "clusters," which cause repeated episodes of intense pain, and headaches resulting from a rise in blood pressure.

Chemical culprits. Repeated exposure to nitrite compounds (such as sodium nitrite, found in hot dogs and other meat products) can result in a dull, pounding headache that may be accompanied by a flushed face.

"Chinese restaurant headache" can occur when a susceptible individual eats foods prepared with monosodium glutamate (MSG)—a staple in many oriental kitchens. Soy sauce, meat tenderizer and a variety of packaged foods contain this chemical, which is touted as a flavor enhancer.

Vascular headache can also result from exposure to poisons, even common household varieties like insecticides, carbon tetrachloride and lead. Painters, printmakers and other artists may experience headaches after exposure to art materials that contain chemicals called solvents. Solvents, like benzene, are found in turpentine, spray adhesives, rubber cement and inks.

Drugs such as amphetamines can cause headaches as a side effect. Another type of drug-related headache occurs during withdrawal from long-term therapy with the antimigraine drug ergotamine tartrate.

A cluster of pain. Cluster headaches, named for their repeated occurrence in groups or clusters, begin as a minor pain around one eye, eventually spreading to that side of the face. The pain quickly intensifies, compelling the victim to pace the floor or rock in a chair. "You can't lie down; you're fidgety," explains a cluster patient. "The pain is unbearable." Other symptoms include a stuffed and runny nose and a droopy eyelid over a red and tearing eye.

Cluster headaches last between 30 and 45 minutes. But the relief people feel at the end of an attack is usually mixed with dread as they await a recurrence. Clusters can strike several times a day or night for several weeks or months. Then, mysteriously, they may disappear for months or years. Many people have cluster bouts during the spring and fall. At their worst, chronic cluster headaches can last continuously for years.

Cluster attacks can strike at any age but usually start between the ages of 20 and 40. Unlike migraine, cluster headaches are more common in men and do not run in families. Research scientists have observed certain physical similarities among people who experience cluster headaches. The typical cluster patient is a tall, muscular man with a rugged facial appearance and a square, jutting or dimpled chin. The texture of his coarse skin resembles an orange peel. Women who get clusters may also have this type of skin.

Studies of cluster patients show that they are likely to have hazel eyes and that they tend to be heavy smokers and drinkers. Paradoxically, both nicotine, which constricts arteries, and alcohol, which dilates them, trigger cluster headaches. The exact connection between these substances and cluster attacks is not known.

Despite a cluster headache's distinguishing characteristics, its relative infrequency and similarity to such disorders as sinusitis can lead to misdiagnosis. Some cluster patients have had tooth extractions, sinus surgery or psychiatric treatment in a futile effort to cure their pain.

Research studies have turned up several clues as to the cause of cluster headaches, but no answers. One clue is found in the thermograms of untreated cluster patients, which show a "cold spot" of reduced blood flow above the eye.

The sudden start and brief duration of cluster headaches can make them difficult to treat. By the time medicine is absorbed into the body, the attack is often over. However, research scientists have identified several effective drugs for these headaches. The antimigraine drug ergotamine tartrate can subdue a cluster if taken at the first sign of an attack. Injections of dihydroergotamine, a form of ergotamine tartrate, are sometimes used to treat clusters. Some cluster patients can prevent attacks by taking propranolol or methysergide.

Another option that works for some cluster patients is rapid inhalation of pure oxygen through a mask for 5 to 15 minutes. The oxygen seems to ease the pain of a cluster headache by reducing blood flow to the brain.

In chronic cases of cluster headache, certain facial nerves may be surgically cut or destroyed to provide relief. These procedures have had limited success. Some cluster patients have had facial nerves cut only to have them regenerate years later.

Painful pressure. Chronic high blood pressure can cause headache, as can rapid rises in blood pressure like those experienced during anger, vigorous exercise or sexual excitement.

The severe "orgasmic headache" occurs right before orgasm and is believed to be a vascular type. Since sudden rupture of a cerebral blood vessel can also occur during orgasm, this type of headache should be promptly evaluated by a doctor.

Muscle-Contraction Headaches: The Everyday Menace

It's 5:00 P.M. and your boss has just asked you to prepare a 20-page briefing paper. Due date: tomorrow. You're angry and tired, and the more you think about the assignment, the tenser you become. Your teeth clench, your brow wrinkles, and soon you have a splitting tension headache.

Tension headache is named not only for the role of stress in triggering the pain but also for the contraction of neck, face and scalp muscles brought on by stressful events. It is a severe but temporary form of muscle-contraction headache. The pain is mild to moderate and feels like pressure is being applied to the head or neck. The headache usually disappears after the period of stress is over.

By contrast, chronic muscle-contraction headaches can last for weeks, months and sometimes years. The pain of these headaches is often described as a tight band around the head or a feeling that the head and neck are in a cast. "It feels like somebody is tightening a giant vise around my head," says one patient. The pain is steady and is usually felt on both sides of the head. Chronic muscle-contraction headaches can cause a sore scalp—even combing one's hair can be painful.

Many scientists believe that the primary cause of the pain of a muscle-contraction headache is sustained muscle tension. Other studies suggest that restricted blood flow may cause or contribute to the pain.

Occasionally, muscle-contraction headaches will be accompanied by nausea, vomiting and blurred vision, but there is no preheadache syndrome such as that which occurs with migraine. Muscle-contraction headaches have not been linked to hormones or foods, as has migraine, nor is there a strong hereditary connection.

Research shows that for many people, chronic muscle-contraction headaches are caused by depression and anxiety. These people tend to get their headaches in the early morning or evening when conflicts in the office or home are anticipated.

Emotional factors are not the only triggers of muscle-contraction headaches. Certain physical postures—such as holding one's chin down while reading—can lead to head and neck pain. Tensing head and neck muscles during sexual excitement can also cause headache. So can prolonged writing under poor light, holding a phone between the shoulder and ear or even gum chewing.

Some more serious problems that can cause muscle-contraction headaches include degenerative arthritis of the neck and temporomandibular joint dysfunction, or TMJ. TMJ is a disorder of the joint between the temporal bone (above the ear) and the mandible, or lower jaw bone. The disorder results from poor bite and jaw clenching.

Treatment for muscle-contraction headache varies. The first consideration is to treat any specific disorder or disease that may be causing the headache. For example, arthritis of the neck is treated with anti-inflammatory medication and TMJ may be helped by corrective devices for the mouth and jaw.

Acute tension headaches not associated with a disease are treated with muscle relaxants and analgesics like aspirin and acetaminophen. Stronger analgesics, such as propoxyphene and codeine, are sometimes prescribed. As prolonged use of these drugs can lead to dependence, patients taking them should have periodic medical checkups and follow their physicians' instructions carefully.

Nondrug therapy for chronic muscle-contraction headaches includes biofeedback, relaxation training and counseling. A technique called cognitive restructuring teaches people to change their attitudes and responses to stress. Patients might be encouraged, for example, to imagine that they are coping successfully with a stressful situation. In progressive relaxation therapy, patients are taught to first tense and then relax individual muscle groups. Finally, the patient tries to relax his or her whole body. Many people imagine a peaceful situation, such as lying on the beach or by a beautiful lake. Passive relaxation does not involve tensing of muscles. Instead, patients are encouraged to focus on different muscles, suggesting that they relax. Some people might think to themselves, "Relax," or "My muscles feel warm."

People with chronic muscle-contraction headaches may also be helped by taking antidepressants or MAO inhibitors. Mixed muscle-contraction and migraine headaches are sometimes treated with barbiturate compounds, which slow down nerve function in the brain and spinal cord.

People who suffer infrequent muscle-contraction headaches may benefit from a hot shower or moist heat applied to the back of the neck. Cervical collars are sometimes recommended to help reduce neck strain. Physical therapy, massage and gentle exercise of the neck may also be helpful.

When Headache Is a Warning

Like other types of pain, headaches can serve as warning signals of more serious disorders. This is particularly true for headaches caused by traction or inflammation.

Traction headaches can occur if the pain-sensitive parts of the head are pulled, stretched or displaced, as, for example, when eye muscles are tensed to compensate for eyestrain. Headaches caused by inflammation include those related to meningitis as well as those resulting from diseases of the sinuses, spine, neck, ears and teeth. Ear and tooth infections and glaucoma can cause headaches. In oral and dental disorders, headache is experienced as pain in the entire head, including the face.

Testing New Treatments

Scientists are developing new therapies and analyzing the effectiveness of current treatment methods for headache. A research team at Southern Illinois University is comparing a biofeedback method that monitors blood flow with a method that monitors muscular tension in the head. This research should lead to improved understanding of individual differences in treatment response.

Several scientists are studying the value of biofeedback and other forms of treatment carried out in the patient's home. Home-based programs may be a boon to patients in rural areas who have limited access to medical care and cannot afford frequent visits to headache specialists.

At the State University of New York in Albany, scientists are comparing the effectiveness of an in-the-doctor's-office relaxation training program for muscle-contraction, migraine and mixed-headache patients with a similar program conducted by patients at home. Patients in the home-based program are seen in the doctor's office once a month but rely heavily on manuals, cassettes and portable biofeedback devices.

Preliminary results suggest that home-based and office-based programs are equally effective. "If these relaxation techniques are learned at home," speculates the investigator, "they may transfer more readily to the home situation—where they will be used to cope with daily stresses."

Furthermore, at the University of Washington in Seattle, an investigator is finding that home-based treatment involving only dietary changes is as effective in treating migraine patients as a home-based program of biofeedback and stress management.

Thermal biofeedback training, which involves the conscious warming of parts of the body through thought control, is believed to work because it gives people a feeling of control over their headaches. A study at Midwest Research Institute in Kansas City, Missouri, raises the possibility that this feeling of control is a more important factor in decreasing headaches than is the actual warming of the hands.

Another important area of research is the study of beta-blocking drugs like propranolol, which are used to prevent migraine.

Beta-blockers stop the activities of beta-receptors—cells in the brain and heart that control the dilation of blood vessels. The ability of beta-blockers to halt the dilation of blood vessels in the brain is believed to be a major reason for their antimigraine action. But because the drugs also affect heart receptors—slowing the heart rate—they cannot be used by people who have certain heart conditions.

PART II:
PROGRESS IN SURGERY

CHAPTER 13
Lasers That Renew Your Heart

Someday soon, doctors may scour out your arteries with scalpels of light.

It's a surgical plumber's snake, this spaghetti-thin strand of optical fibers shimmying up an artery in your arm, twisting and bending as it follows a circuitous path into your coronary arteries.

From the tip of the flexible catheter, a ghostly ribbon of light fires at the debris-laden artery walls. In a series of bursts, this miniature light saber blasts away even the most hardened fat and cholesterol deposits lining the blood vessels.

When the procedure is over, the probe is safely withdrawn through a small slit in your arm, and the muck and mire that took half a lifetime to accumulate is gone. Your arteries have been scoured as clean as a soda straw, and blood is pulsing through a clear channel for the first time since you were born.

No, you haven't beamed aboard the Starship Enterprise. But you have traveled just a few years into the future of heart surgery.

This space-age surgical technique is called percutaneous laser angioplasty, meaning a laser delivered under the skin by a flexible tube or catheter. Right now, percutaneous laser angioplasty is undergoing tests in research centers across the nation. But within the next few years, these high-powered surgical lasers may find their way into your heart.

So far, the technique has been attempted only on the blood vessels of cadavers (dead bodies) and has also been employed to open blocked arteries in legs. But if the new laser technology works, thousands of people who would otherwise be candidates for a coronary bypass operation will be spared the expense, the emotional trauma and the physical disability of this highly invasive surgery.

An even more intriguing possibility, however, is that laser angioplasty may someday be used to control atherosclerosis (hardening of the arteries due to fat and cholesterol buildup) well before it becomes a life-threatening problem.

"It should be feasible for otherwise perfectly well people to get laser treatment for, say, a 40 or 50 percent narrowing of the coronary arteries, many years before problems would begin," according to Kenneth I. Shine, M.D., dean of the UCLA School of Medicine and president of the American Heart Association. "I think you'll see it happen before the end of this decade."

High-Tech Hardware

Crafting such a precise surgical tool calls for an unusual wedding of traditional medical science with high technology. At California's Cedars-Sinai Medical Center, an unlikely team of surgeons, NASA scientists and optical engineers has developed just such a device.

Surgeons at Cedars-Sinai have been experimenting with a variety of lasers for the past few years. But they hadn't found one that would fill the bill until they read news of a precise, high-powered xenon-chloride excimer laser developed by physicists at NASA's Jet Propulsion Laboratory under James B. Laudenslager, Ph.D.

The word excimer is scientific shorthand for "excited dimer." Two gases—xenon and chloride—are "excited" by an electrical discharge. The two gases together constitute a dimer, a union of molecules from two elements.

The excited atoms of xenon-chloride bounce back and forth in a mirrored tube, colliding with the subatomic building blocks of light called photons and producing a needle-sharp strand of ultraviolet light that is allowed to escape out one end of the tube.

Using magnetic switches, the light of the excimer is switched on and off in pulses lasting a hundred-millionth of a second. This feature makes the excimer well suited to the problem of clearing away arterial debris without french-frying the artery wall.

"One of the reasons we use a pulsed ultraviolet laser is that ultraviolet light doesn't penetrate tissue very deeply," says Dr. Laudenslager. "It's kind of like setting up a drill press to drill a small hole a quarter-inch deep. Set up the drill press once, and it won't go any deeper than a quarter-inch or wider than a drill bit. Each pulse will remove a certain, predetermined area with a certain thickness. It won't go any deeper or wider. The same principle applies to the excimer."

Because the excimer carves out a preset niche for itself with every pulse, it obliterates only what it touches, one thin layer at a time. In early tests, the excimer has sliced through coronary plaque without burning or scarring tender artery walls. Since scarring may give plaque a place to take root, this kind of control is essential.

"When you're trying to remove a blockage in a blood vessel that's only 1 to 1½ millimeters in diameter [less than 1⁄10 of an inch], you don't want to heat it," Dr. Laudenslager says. "You just want a very clean cut."

Adapting the excimer to use in the heart was one thing. Developing a steerable probe that would carry the beam all the way into the body without disintegrating was quite another. Competing researchers in the red-hot race to develop the perfect heart laser doubted it could be done.

After almost two years of study by Tsvi Goldenberg, Ph.D., an engineer at AT&T Bell Labs, however, Cedars-

Sinai surgeons believe they now have a fiberoptic tough enough to bear up under the excimer's powerful beam yet flexible enough to shimmy into narrow blood vessels. The flexible tubing would also carry lenses to give doctors a clear inside view of the clogged channels.

Is Laser Top Gun?

Despite the optimism, some questions still remain. For instance, will laser-blasted bits of plaque break off and lodge in an artery, causing a heart attack or stroke? Will the arteries remain open?

Critics also wonder whether lasers will ever compete with coronary bypass surgery, in which veins from a patient's leg are removed and used to replace diseased coronary arteries. And they question whether lasers are any better at clearing clogged blood vessels than one currently popular and often successful technique, balloon angioplasty. Instead of blasting plaque, a tiny balloon probe is threaded into the arteries to the area of blockage. Then the balloon is inflated several times with a liquid, opening a passage by flattening the debris against blood-vessel walls.

Dr. Shine doesn't think these questions are without answers. "Assuming these problems can be resolved, laser angioplasty will compete with bypass surgery for a number of patients.

"Right now, 20 to 30 percent of all patients who once would have been candidates for bypass surgery are instead going for balloon angioplasty," says Dr. Shine. "Even if the laser simply doubled that percentage, you'd be reducing the need for surgery by half."

Laser probes might also someday work in partnership with balloon angioplasty. One of the main drawbacks of the balloon is its inability to penetrate hardened, or calcified, plaque. But the laser can cut through a blockage like an icebreaker, leaving clear passage for the balloon. Such a technique is being developed by doctors at the Boston University Medical Center.

No matter who wins the race to develop the safest, most potent plaque-buster, laser angioplasty is likely to pose some risks. No one can be certain what those risks might be. But, says Dr. Shine, "There are going to be problems with anything you do. There are always risks when you put catheters into blood vessels."

Still, lasers are likely to remain on the cutting edge of surgical technology. "The most exciting thing," says Dr. Shine, "is how one technology has led to another. When balloon angioplasty started, that led to the development of steerable catheters. And now, because of steerable catheters, it becomes much more feasible to think about using a laser in man."

CHAPTER 14

Stroke-Prevention Surgery: How Safe Is It?

New research takes a provocative look at the risks and benefits of this popular operation.

Take your hand and feel the pulse in your neck. That artery, the carotid, is your main lifeline. Your life depends on an adequate supply of the oxygen in your blood getting through this artery to your brain from minute to minute.

A doctor could put a stethoscope to your neck and tell you whether the artery is becoming clogged with fatty buildup due to atherosclerosis. He would hear a bruit (pronounced *brew-ee*), which is the sound of blood rushing through a narrowed artery. You may not feel ill, but a bruit signals that something's wrong. If you have a bruit, your chances of having a stroke almost double.

An operation called a carotid endarterectomy opens up and cleans out the carotid artery. It has become the most widely performed noncardiac vascular surgery in the United States, and its popularity is increasing rapidly. There was a 74 percent increase in the number of these operations performed between 1980 and 1984.

But while most doctors believe that carotid endarterectomies help prevent strokes, researchers are now finding that those who have bruits but no other warning signs of stroke may be better off without the operation.

Researchers at the Cincinnati College of Medicine looked at the results of 1,181 carotid endarterectomies performed over the course of a year. They found the stroke and death rate associated with the procedure "alarming" and expressed concern that carotid endarterectomies are being performed too frequently.

Of the asymptomatic people (those with only bruits but no other real symptoms), 5.3 percent either had a stroke or died during surgery or shortly afterward. The majority of injuries resulting from strokes were permanent. That amount was considerably higher than the 3 percent that has been suggested as reasonable for "prophylactic" carotid surgery.

Since half of all endarterectomies are being performed on asymptomatic people, that means there may be more than 1,000 unnecessary deaths and even more unnecessary strokes this year as a result of the surgery.

The Cincinnati researchers are not sure whether the procedure is any better than treating patients with aspirin or other drugs. They do suggest, however, that for asymptomatic patients "a more conservative approach is warranted" until further evidence supports the therapeutic value of the surgery (*Journal of the American Medical Association*).

"The purpose of our study was to find out what was actually being achieved today in a representative metropolitan community. Then we can focus our decision making in a more realistic light," says one of the researchers, Richard F. Kempczinski, M.D., a vascular surgeon at the University of Cincinnati College of Medicine.

"As I review the literature and the studies to date, it seems to me that asymptomatic patients are at greater risk because of the surgery than if they didn't have it. But not everyone interprets this the same way," says Mark Dyken, M.D., professor and chairman of the Department of Neurology at the Indiana School of Medicine and chairman of the American Heart Association's Stroke Council. "There are a lot of people over age 50 who have varying degrees of atherosclerosis. We know that disease is a risk for stroke, but all the evidence we have is that it's a random risk. It's not directly or closely related to the vessels involved in surgery."

How Strokes Develop

Atherosclerosis is the instigator behind most strokes. The linings of the arteries become thickened by deposits of fat, cholesterol, fibrin (a clotting material), dead cells and calcium. Blood flows through the arteries and veins but tends to clot when it comes in contact with this "garbage," which is politely called plaque. The plaque may be marked with little craters. These craters can give rise to clots. A blood clot or a piece of the plaque may break off and travel to the brain, causing a stroke.

When that happens, the brain is deprived of oxygen and part of the brain may die. Depending on where the damage occurs, you may develop paralysis or lose your speech, hearing, sight or the ability to swallow. Usually when they're gone, they're gone for good.

The carotid arteries are prime targets for blockages because atherosclerotic buildup occurs most often where vessels narrow and branch off. In your neck, you have two carotid arteries—one on each side—each of which divides into two more arteries, the external carotid and the internal carotid. The external carotid branches off to your head and neck, while the internal carotid shoots up to the brain, the optic nerve and retina, passing onto and through a traffic circle in the base of the skull. Both carotids contribute to this circle, which works as a communicating system so that if one artery is blocked, the others may help out.

Through further tests, most using ultrasound, a doctor can get a better idea of the size and location of the blockage in the carotid. The reduction in the diameter of the vessel is labeled minimal when it is 10 to 15 percent closed, moderate at 16 to 49 percent and severe at 50 to 99 percent.

Before surgery, digital intravenous angiography (DIVA) is performed. This test may have some risks because it involves injecting dye into a vein, but it is highly accurate. An image is created from x-rays taken at different times and stored on a computer. These images combined give an even clearer picture of the extent of the blockage, and surgeons use it like a road map.

During the operation, the carotid artery is opened, and the plaque is carefully scraped out. Some surgeons may prefer to use local anesthesia so the patient can report numbness or weakness when the carotid is clamped. Others prefer general anesthesia.

Does Anyone Benefit?

In light of these new findings, who would still benefit from a carotid endarterectomy?

"This is where you come into a gray area," says Howard C. Baron, M.D., attending vascular surgeon at Cabrini Medical Center and a practicing vascular surgeon in New York. "I feel that if there is a bruit in each artery, this is dangerous, and that person would be operated on. Not simultaneously, but in stages over a period of time. If, in any asymptomatic patient, you find a bruit only on one side that occupies more than 50 percent of the diameter of the internal carotid, that patient is a candidate for surgery and should go through the usual diagnostic procedures. If you don't operate, two to five years from now the person may have other systemic diseases, and he becomes a poorer surgical risk."

"If the artery is starting to occlude, then clearly you would be better off if somebody could go in there and open it up," says Dr. Kempczinski. "Unfortunately, no surgeon operates without a certain degree of complication, and therefore the decision to proceed with surgery or not to proceed with surgery is a careful balance between the risk of an operation versus the risk of conventional medical treatment.

"For asymptomatic patients, we really don't know the risks and benefits of conventional treatment at the present time," he adds. "If I fell in that category, then I would consent to an angiogram to determine and confirm the noninvasive study. If that angiogram showed that I had a tight narrowing of over 80 percent, I'd find myself a good surgeon and get it fixed."

Other doctors feel strongly that the consequences of the surgery are more dangerous than the operation. "I don't have any of my asymptomatic patients operated on," says Dr. Dyken.

The proper studies haven't been done to find out who is better off with the operation, with medical treatment or with no treatment. A more definitive answer may be available five to seven years down the road. "In the meantime, I think we have to be conservative," Dr. Dyken stresses.

The answer would differ, however, for patients with symptoms who have not been helped by medical therapy. "It seems logical to me that if you have a surgeon who has a very low complication rate, those people would be candidates for surgery," adds Dr. Dyken.

Symptoms of Artery Blockage

Symptoms, often produced by episodes called transient ischemic attacks (TIAs), include feelings of numbness or weakness in the face, arm or leg on one side, difficulty speaking, memory lapses or temporary blindness. The blindness, which usually affects just one eye, has been described by patients as having a curtain pulled down over their eye. The sight gradually clears. They may also have dizziness or double vision or stagger while walking.

TIAs usually last from 30 seconds to 3 minutes. Almost all clear within 30 minutes. A person may have only a few attacks or several hundred. A stroke may occur after only one or two attacks or after a hundred have occurred over a period of weeks or months. Sometimes the attacks gradually cease.

If surgery is the appropriate choice, patients should ask a neurologist in their area for the name of a good surgeon who is getting excellent results with carotid endarterectomies, Dr. Kempczinski suggests. In addition, a list of doctors in your area who specialize in carotid endarterectomies may be obtained from your local medical society. And don't hesitate to ask several doctors and patients for recommendations.

When surgery is not called for, there are several alternatives. Some blockages in the carotid may just be checked periodically, and others can be treated medically with anticlotting drugs or aspirin to keep the blood flowing freely.

Many researchers think that the death rate from stroke has declined in recent years because high blood pressure is now being controlled more effectively. High blood pressure, in fact, is one of the greatest risk factors for stroke. You may also reduce your risk of having a stroke by controlling diabetes, eating a low-fat diet, exercising regularly, not drinking excessively and not smoking.

CHAPTER 15

Vasectomy Reversal: The Odds Get Better

Microsurgery is now helping to turn sterilized men into new fathers.

In the old days (say, 15 years ago), once you decided to get off the reproductive merry-go-round by having a vasectomy, the party was over for good. You were *permanently* sterilized. And if later in life—say, after remarriage to a younger woman—you suddenly began to long for the sound of a baby's wail, well, you and your wife could either adopt a child, rent a record or move next door to a baby.

Today that reality has dramatically changed. If you had a vasectomy even as long as 10 or 20 years ago and now wish you hadn't, a skilled microsurgeon stands roughly a 90 percent chance of being able to restore your fertility.

This was the heartening news in the numbers presented by Sherman Silber, M.D., a reproductive microsurgeon at St. Luke's West Hospital in St. Louis, at a meeting of the American Urological Association. Over a period of ten years, Dr. Silber has performed 3,000 vasectomy reversals. The decade-long follow-up on these men has shown that over three-quarters of them have since become fathers.

Considering the difficulty of the operation, this record is a testament to impressively steady hands and advanced microsurgical technique. A vasectomy is a relatively simple, 15-minute operation in which the vas deferens—the tiny tube that carries sperm from the testicles out into the world—is snipped in two, thus neatly interrupting a man's fertility. The reversal operation, on the other hand, involves stitching the vas deferens back together again—we're talking here about a vessel whose walls are a thousandth of an inch thick and whose inner diameter is narrower than a human hair. The operation may take anywhere from 1½ to 5 hours, depending on the surgeon's skill, and it costs about as much as a decent used car (upwards of $6,000, not all of which is covered by health insurance). But if you want to become a father badly enough, it may well be worth the price.

In the case of men whose vasectomies caused no damage to the epididymis (the very delicate sperm storage duct that conveys sperm from the testicle into the vas deferens), 99 percent showed normal sperm counts after the reversal operation, Dr. Silber reports. And the pregnancy rate for the wives of these men hit 88.9 percent. "That's really exciting, because that's about the same as you'd expect in a normal population," he says.

Among the men whose vasectomies did cause some damage to the epididymis, Dr. Silber reports, the reversal operation restored normal sperm counts in 89 percent. After seven years of follow-up, there was also a 79 percent pregnancy rate among their wives.

Normally, between the time sperm is manufactured in the testes and the time it is eventually expelled out of the body through the vas deferens, it's stored in the epididymis, a 20-foot-long tube that's coiled up into a space about an inch long, Dr. Silber explains. But after the vas deferens is severed in a vasectomy, there's a gradual buildup of pressure in this fragile duct system. Eventually, this pressure can cause a rupture or blowout, which is sometimes painful. About 30 percent of men who had their operation five years ago have had some epididymal damage, he says. Among men whose operation was performed ten or more years ago, about 70 percent show some damage. If there have been epididymal blowouts caused by this pressure increase, the area of blockage in the epididymis must also be bypassed. If only the vas deferens is reconnected, the operation will still fail because of blockage closer to the testicle.

The bottom line: The longer it has been since you had your vasectomy, the more likely it is that you've had some epididymal damage—which will make the reversal operation much more difficult. But in the hands of an experienced microsurgeon, the chances of success can still be quite good.

PART III: NEW HOPE WITH BETTER DRUG TREATMENTS

CHAPTER 16

Wielding the Power of Arthritis Drugs

New anti-inflammatory medications are bringing welcome relief to many. But the risks must be weighed carefully.

The two faces of arthritis medications—the visages of help and harm—prompt pointed questions: Do the drugs' benefits outweigh their risks? Which ones are the most effective? Can they do anything more than simply suppress symptoms? Exactly how do they work?

Finding the answers means putting the sword to myths that are as old as the drugs themselves.

Myth #1: Arthritis medications are simple substances with the simple function of killing pain. With over 100 enigmatic forms, arthritis itself isn't a simple disease, and the drugs used to treat it have matching complexity.

For one thing, anti-arthritis agents aren't just painkillers or analgesics, though they may contain some analgesic component. Usually, numbing the pain—and *only* numbing the pain—isn't entirely the point. Most serious forms of arthritis are basically an inflammation of tissue, most likely a joint. This means pain, all right, but also swelling, redness, heat, stiffness and even damage to the tissue. So the idea is to reverse the inflammation, reducing all its symptoms (including pain) in the process. Thus, like aspirin (the most prescribed arthritis medication in America), most arthritis drugs are primarily anti-inflammatories. Through intricate processes that scientists are still arguing over, these substances try to cool inflamed joint tissue, the core symptom of the nation's number one crippling disease.

Arthritis experts have drawn clear distinctions between such anti-inflammatories and popular painkillers like Tylenol, Darvon, Demerol and others. James F. Fries, M.D., director of the Stanford University Arthritis Clinic and author of *Arthritis: A Comprehensive Guide,* says that painkillers have little place in arthritis therapy.

"First," he says, "they don't do anything for the arthritis; they just cover it up. Second, they help defeat the pain mechanism that tells you when you are doing something that is injuring your body. Third, the body adjusts to pain medicines, so they aren't very effective over the long term. This phenomenon is called tolerance, and it develops to some extent with all of the drugs we commonly use. Fourth, pain medicines can have major side effects."

But then side effects are some of the things that complicate arthritis drugs. They remind us that the drugs are complex blends of healing power and malevolent potential. Doctors don't even talk about selecting arthritis medications with few side effects, for the drugs average 30 or 40 possible adverse reactions apiece. Physicians speak of balancing the dosage that gives the most relief against the dosage that risks the most toxicity.

"Because of possible drug reactions, patients need to make sure they're taking the medication appropriately," says Paul H. Waytz, M.D., a Minneapolis rheumatologist. "And they need to alert their doctor to any problems. If they're this careful, side effects can be kept to a minimum and are usually reversible."

Myth #2: Arthritis drugs are ultimate solutions to arthritis. By now most arthritis sufferers know that drugs are not "magic bullets" that can kill arthritis forever. For, as arthritis experts keep insisting, the disease isn't curable like pneumonia or appendicitis. "With drugs we can control most signs and symptoms of arthritis," says Dr. Waytz. "We may even be able to force some forms of arthritis into remission. But we may not be able to completely eradicate the disease."

But neither is there an unshakable guarantee that the drugs can always completely manage symptoms. Like arthritis sufferer Louise Patrick, people sometimes discover that arthritis medications don't always live up to their expectations. "I assumed that the drugs would somehow take away the pain, so I'd never again be bothered with it," she says. "But that hasn't happened. My system eventually gets used to the medicine, and the pain slowly returns."

At any rate, doctors point out that the drugs were never meant to be anyone's sole defense against arthritis. "There's a danger in assuming that anti-arthritis compounds should be the answer to your disease," says Robert S. Mendelsohn, M.D., president of the New Medical Foundation in Chicago. "The attitude precludes nondrug therapies that have proven very effective."

Myth #3: An arthritis drug is equally effective for everyone with the same type of arthritis. Arthritics who believe this can end up scratching their head when they compare notes with a fellow arthritis sufferer. Someone with rheumatoid arthritis (RA) may get relief with Motrin; another RA victim may not. Somebody with osteoarthritis may think Indocin is strong medicine; another afflicted with the same disease may say Indocin isn't strong enough. The wide variations in the way people respond to arthritis medications are a matter of scientific record.

"This lack of predictability in response is something that arthritics have to adjust to," says George Ehrlich, M.D., rheumatologist and adjunct professor of medicine at New York University School of Medicine. "They have to be patient, for a doctor may need to switch them from one medication to another to find one that's effective."

And the medicinal options are many. There are over a hundred anti-arthritis drugs around, many of them experimental and some of them as familiar to arthritics as table salt. They're a pharmaceutical spectrum that ranges from lifesaving substance to medicinal reject. Here's a report card on the major categories.

The Number One Medicine

Despite the recent appearance of upstart arthritis medications, the cheapest and most widely used anti-arthritis preparation is still aspirin. Most rheumatologists recommend this ancient medicine (technically acetylsalicylic acid) as a first-line defense against arthritis before trying the younger, high-tech concoctions. And even now it's frequently the yardstick by which other arthritis drugs are measured. Doctors prescribe it by the carload for several forms of arthritis, including osteoarthritis, juvenile arthritis and RA.

People who suffer from these, however, may be looking for different effects from aspirin. Some (like many osteoarthritis patients) may be after the mild analgesic component. Others (like those with RA) may need the potent anti-inflammatory response. But getting what you want means calibrating dosages.

Dr. Fries believes that the strictly analgesic effect of aspirin is at its maximum after two tablets (ten grains) and lasts about four hours. "In contrast," he says, "the anti-inflammatory activity requires high and sustained blood levels of the aspirin. A patient must take 12 to 24 tablets (five grains each) each day, and the process must be continued for weeks to obtain the full effect." Such a regimen is standard therapy for RA sufferers and requires lots of medical supervision.

But often even a watchful physician can't avert what has frequently become headline news: aspirin's side effects. They range from mild to severe and occur in at least 30 percent of arthritics using the drug. Aspirin-takers have had to contend with peptic ulcers, upset stomach, stomach bleeding, tinnitus (ringing in the ears), hearing loss, liver damage and even interference with the blood's ability to clot. On top of all that, aspirin is, next to penicillin, the drug most likely to cause an allergic reaction.

Many doctors argue, however, that you can avoid much of the gastrointestinal havoc by taking aspirin with food or by using either coated aspirin or substances called the nonacetylated salicylates, which are almost identical to aspirin. (These are not the same as the substance found in nonaspirin compounds like Tylenol.)

The New Anti-Inflammatories

The search for arthritis medications that are as effective as aspirin but less toxic led researchers to nonsteroidal anti-inflammatory drugs (NSAIDs). They're a handful of chemically diverse substances sporting brand names that arthritis victims have been hearing for years—Motrin, Indocin, Nalfon, Clinoril, Naprosyn, Butazolidin, Tolectin and others. They all have some analgesic potential and roughly as much anti-inflammatory power as aspirin; they may therefore have the ability to prevent inflammatory damage. Whatever types of arthritis yield to aspirin yield also to NSAIDs.

But the similarities stop there. For one thing, these drugs, though more expensive than aspirin, generally require an RA sufferer to take fewer pills. A person with RA may need to take only 2 Naprosyn tablets a day, but 15 aspirin. Doctors and patients both know that the fewer pills you must contend with, the more likely you are to stick with a dosage schedule.

And though NSAIDs cause most of the same side effects that aspirin does, the reactions are generally less severe. In fact, because of its safety record, one NSAID, ibuprofen, sold by prescription as Motrin and Rufen, earned over-the-counter analgesic status as Advil, Nuprin and other brands.

Some doctors, however, caution that it's too early to hail NSAIDs as safer alternatives to aspirin. "Aspirin has been used for centuries," says Dr. Fries, "whereas experience with these new drugs is sufficiently limited that some side effects may not yet have been discovered."

Then there are those few NSAIDs that are giving the others a bad name. Oraflex and Zomax were removed from the market because they were associated with deaths. And the serious side effects caused by phenylbutazone (Butazolidin) and indomethacin (Indocin) have raised grave doubts about their use.

An American Medical Association (AMA) guide to medications says that phenylbutazone can cause jaundice, hepatitis, blood in the urine, edema, rashes, gastrointestinal disturbances and—worst of all—bone marrow toxicity. Such toxicity can lead to aplastic anemia, a condition that's often fatal.

Indocin's possible adverse reactions may be even more disturbing. It shares many of phenylbutazone's possible side effects (including bone marrow toxicity) and causes some bizarre reactions of its own: eye disturbances, kidney trouble, confusion, coma and even behavioral problems. Perhaps most worrisome of all are the possible ulcerations of the esophagus, stomach and small intestine. Regarding this problem, the AMA says that perforation and hemorrhage (sometimes fatal) have been reported.

The Steroids

In the 1950s, these substances took the medical world by storm, drawing enthusiastic praise from doctors and patients alike, capturing the unofficial titles of "wonder drugs" and "miracle medicines." And, indeed, cortisone—the first of the steroid drugs—had actually enabled RA cripples to walk, run and even jump—free of pain.

But then reality set in, says J. T. Scott, M.D., consulting physician at Charing Cross Hospital in London and author of *Arthritis and Rheumatism: The Facts.* It soon became clear, he says, that "the dosage of cortisone required to suppress the disease—and it did more than that—produced also an alarming concatenation of toxic effects, ranging from the unsightly and hairy 'moon face' to perforating and bleeding gastric ulceration." And now, 30 years after the steroid debut, doctors are still wielding this medicinal two-edged sword—but more gingerly.

Corticosteroids are hormones manufactured by the adrenal glands, and when the body gets an extra dose of the compounds (by injection of cortisone or prednisone, for example), inflammatory symptoms can be dampened dramatically. NSAIDs or aspirin simply can't match this anti-inflammatory vigor.

Nowadays, what doctors try to do in steroid therapy is walk the thin line between this positive force and side effects like ulcers, skin disorders, bone disease and cataracts. And they do this by carefully controlling dosages and duration of treatment. Taking low-dose steroids for a short term or getting a single injection in a troublesome joint isn't likely to cause severe reactions in the properly selected patient. But long-term, high-dose steroid treatment is practically guaranteed to cause health problems worse than arthritis itself.

"In certain cases of RA, steroids can actually be lifesaving," says Sanford H. Roth, M.D., Phoenix rheumatologist and editor of *Handbook of Drug Therapy in Rheumatology*. "And low-dose steroids can be useful in select situations. But generally, if we can achieve good results without steroids, we should not use them because of the many problems common to long-term hormonal therapy."

The Remission-Inducing Drugs

These chemically unrelated compounds are the big guns of arthritis drug therapy—mighty medicines that can suppress symptoms for long periods, even bully disease into remission. They originally were used to treat diseases other than arthritis, but now they're used primarily for RA patients who have failed to respond to other drugs. And, like all arthritis medications, they have their risks.

Gold salts (Solganal, Myochrysine and Ridaura) are probably the most popular remission-inducing compounds among both rheumatologists and patients. They seem to work for about 75 percent of RA patients who try them, and some people achieve such deep remissions that neither doctor nor patient can detect the disease. But it can take weeks for the therapy to start working. Once it does, however, the beneficial effects can last for months, long after the treatment is stopped.

How do these agents work? No one knows. They certainly exert an anti-inflammatory force, but scientists have yet to figure out why. How did anybody discover that the world's most precious metal has such therapeutic power? Accidentally. Years ago doctors thought RA was caused by tuberculosis (TB) germs, and since gold was being used to treat TB, they decided to try it out on RA patients. And it worked. It wasn't until later, though, that physicians learned—as they did with cortisone—that there was a physical price to pay for success.

Now we know that about 30 percent of those who receive gold treatments will experience side effects—most of them mild but some of them life-threatening. Medical reports mention possible skin rashes, jaundice, mouth ulcers, kidney damage, blood disorders and aplastic anemia.

"Because of the potential problems, patients taking gold have to be carefully monitored," says Dr. Waytz. "They should have periodic urine tests and blood counts. And at the first sign of adverse reactions, the drug should be withdrawn."

All of which goes double for another remission-inducing drug called penicillamine. This by-product of the manufacture of penicillin has much in common with gold but has more potential for harm. Like gold, its workings are mysterious, long-term and impressively effective (50 to 60 percent of patients will get some relief). But it has most of gold's possible side effects plus a few more: gastrointestinal disturbances, autoimmune disease, taste impairment, explosive vomiting and fatal bone marrow disruption. Some of these will occur in 40 to 50 percent of those who take the drug.

"Penicillamine," says Dr. Waytz, "should be administered in the lowest possible dose that will suppress the signs and symptoms of rheumatoid arthritis."

The antimalarial compounds, on the other hand, aren't nearly as toxic as gold or penicillamine, but then they're probably not as effective, either. They're derivatives of quinine, a medication used around the world to combat malaria. Doctors don't know exactly how yet, but these agents (chloroquine and hydroxychloroquine) can offer relief to victims of several inflammatory diseases, including RA. It may take three to six months for the drugs to work, but the positive effects could last just as long.

Using the medications for such lengthy periods, though, is bound to cause some problems. Skin rashes, sores, gastrointestinal disturbances, hair blanching—these are the occasional and reversible penalties. A rare and possibly irreversible one is far more serious: blindness.

Doctors now are also using cancer drugs, including Methotrexate and azathioprine (Imuran), to fight RA. These drugs can slow the progress of RA and help control it. Although serious side effects may occur, arthritis patients receive much smaller dosages than those used in treating cancer. Physicians closely monitor these patients for such side effects as bone marrow or liver toxicity and can alter treatment before problems develop.

Weighing risks against benefits is the arthritis sufferer's lot—a serious business that requires a respect for medicinal power and a need for straight answers.

One arthritis sufferer, Christiaan Barnard, M.D., preeminent surgeon and author of *Christiaan Barnard's Program for Living with Arthritis,* offers this advice: "Ask as many questions as you can about the length of time you will need to take the tablets offered, how they act, what their side effects are, what their dangers and potential benefits are. If the drug is newly developed, ask your doctor whether it genuinely offers something that other compounds already tried and tested on the market cannot provide. Play for safety, not spectacular overnight results. There are no miracles in medicine. Superb, marvelous treatments, but no miracles."

CHAPTER 17

High-Tech Healing: Medicine in a Patch

Innovative devices that send medicine through the skin are making treatment easier and more effective than ever.

Here's something you may experience soon, if you haven't already: high-tech Band-Aid-like patches that deliver medication through the skin. Instead of having to remember to take a pill every four hours or so, you have only to remember to change your patch every day, every three days or once a week.

These patches are currently available to prevent motion sickness, angina and high blood pressure. Look for one soon that will deliver estrogen, a medication many women take to prevent the side effects of menopause, such as hot flashes, mood swings and osteoporosis. Others are being developed and tested that may revolutionize forever the way many of us take medications.

Direct Delivery

Until recently, scientists thought the skin to be a more impenetrable barrier than it really is. A typical square inch of skin contains 50 hair follicles, 60 nerves, 75 sebaceous glands and 500 sweat glands. Underneath, networks of capillaries feed into the bloodstream. The drugs in a patch make their way through the tough but thin outer layer and inner layers of skin and fat and then are absorbed directly into the bloodstream.

When you take a pill, the medication must go through your stomach, intestines and liver before making its way into your bloodstream. Because the liver inactivates many drugs, a large dose must be given to achieve the desired therapeutic effect. It's like using a fire hose to put out a candle. With the patch, less medication can give the same therapeutic effects, which often results in fewer side effects.

Soon after you take a pill, the medication in your blood peaks, then it gradually drops off, and you need to take another pill. That cycle often repeats several times a day. On top of that, many of us forget to take medicine. A patch releases its dose at an even rate, keeping the level of medication in your blood steady; it's easy to apply, and you are supposed to forget about it temporarily. If you have a problem, you simply remove the patch. When you take a pill, once you swallow it, you have little control over what happens.

Patches differ slightly, but basically they are constructed in four thin layers: an impermeable backing, a minute drug reservoir, a membrane that controls the release rate of the drug and an adhesive layer that is attached to a peel-off backing.

The patch delivers medicine as though you were receiving an IV, but without a needle. As soon as you apply a patch, the drug begins flowing through the skin into the blood at a rate regulated by the membrane. There is usually a priming dose in the adhesive layer to help raise the drug level in the blood to therapeutic levels more quickly.

Patches on the Market

Here are the patches that are currently available.

Clonidine (CATAPRES TTS). This drug for high blood pressure has been available in a patch since September, 1985. You put the patch on the upper part of the body—either the chest or the upper arm—and leave it on for a full week. This may be its most important benefit, since many people with high blood pressure don't feel sick, and they often forget to take their medicine. The patch stays on during swimming, showering or exercising. If it should begin to peel at the edges, it comes with an overlay patch to put over it for the rest of the week. The patch comes in different sizes for different dosages.

"In mild hypertension where the diastolic blood pressure (the bottom number) is less than 105, about 70 to 75 percent of patients are getting normal blood pressure just with the patch alone," says Mark Houston, M.D., assistant professor of medicine and co-director of the medical intensive care unit at Vanderbilt University Medical Center in Nashville.

Dr. Houston has conducted clinical studies on the patch and clonidine for several years. "Other patients may require a second medication like a low dose of a diuretic or something else," he says. "The patients who have more severe high blood pressure obviously require more medication, not only through the patch but orally as well."

"Clonidine, whether given through the skin patch or in pill form, works very much the same and is effective in decreasing blood pressure in hypertensive patients," says Michael Weber, M.D., professor of medicine and chief of clinical pharmacology and hypertension at the University of California-Irvine College of Medicine. Dr. Weber conducted clinical trials of the patch. "A big difference was that side effects were far less on the patch. Complaints like dry mouth, drowsiness or headaches were far fewer. We think the main reason for that is that when you give clonidine transdermally [through the skin], you get the same antihypertensive effect with only about half as much drug.

"People taking other kinds of drugs who are having side effects or other problems have found switching to the patch to be a big step forward," says Dr. Weber. "Some people like it because it's convenient. You have to apply it only once a week. The patients who are on it often love it. They are its greatest advocates.

"About 10 to 20 percent get some type of skin reaction to the patch, however, and about half of those might have to stop using it," he says. Some people get redness or itching under the patch. In some instances this can be severe, but usually it's a very mild nuisance that doesn't cause any real concern. Rotating the patch from one area to another decreases the chances of that.

Two other side effects are sometimes seen. Mild sedation occurs about 25 percent of the time but tends to go away after a month or two. Dry mouth may occur, but it also tends to go away with time, says Dr. Houston.

Rebound hypertension, found when oral medication is stopped, has not been noted in those who stop using the patch. This might be because when the patch is removed, blood levels of the medication fall slowly.

Scopolamine (Transderm-Scop). This drug, for motion sickness, was the first drug available in patch form. Scopolamine is a very effective drug for motion sickness. But in the high dosages necessary when given orally or injected, it causes unacceptable side effects.

Now you can just place the dime-size patch behind your ear about four hours before you get on a boat or plane. The drug is absorbed into the bloodstream and prevents the fatigue, nausea and malaise that go along with motion sickness. One patch lasts for three days. If you're on a cruise for six days, you take it off one ear and put a new one on the other ear right away. The patch, available only by prescription, is especially handy if you're nauseated and can't swallow a pill and keep it down.

There are still some side effects to watch out for. About two out of three people experience dry mouth. One out of six gets drowsy, but the patch doesn't cause drowsiness as often as other motion-sickness medicines. Rarely, users have experienced confusion, agitation, hallucinations, insomnia, blurred vision and dilation of the pupils in the eyes. These problems are all reversible, however, by removing the patch.

Nitroglycerin (Transderm-Nitro, Nitro-Dur and Nitrodisc). This is a drug for angina, which occurs when a coronary artery is narrowed and the heart, which has been stimulated by exercise, excitement or anxiety, demands more blood than it can get. Nitroglycerin, when taken sublingually (under the tongue), heads right into the bloodstream and widens the blood vessels in seconds. This is similar to transdermal delivery. The patch, however, lasts 24 hours and is used to prevent angina before it happens.

Before the patch was available, most people took multiple daily doses of nitroglycerin tablets or capsules or applied an ointment several times a day to prevent angina attacks. But nitroglycerin when swallowed isn't very effective because the liver metabolizes all of the drug almost immediately. And you have to measure the nitroglycerin ointment from a tube and spread it on the skin several times a day. (This works the same as the patch, but it's messy and the dosage is difficult to control.)

Different brands of the patch are available; they can be worn anywhere on the body except below the knees and elbows, but they work best when placed on the chest or back. They are now smaller and easier to wear than when they were first introduced.

Recently, researchers evaluated the effectiveness of nitroglycerin patches. They found that while the effects of nitroglycerin may vary from patient to patient, the patches frequently increase exercise time. The patches also lowered the incidence of hospitalization and emergency room visits. And the researchers found that most patients prefer the patch over the oral medication or ointment.

Estrogen (Estraderm). This patch, to relieve the symptoms of menopause, was recently approved by the U.S. Food and Drug Administration (FDA). Usually worn on the abdomen, the patch lasts 3½ days.

Twenty-three postmenopausal women tested the patch at UCLA. Researchers found that the estrogen, by bypassing the liver, did not—as oral estrogen does—increase the level of liver proteins that can increase the risk of high blood pressure. The patch, like oral estrogen, also reduced calcium loss through the urine, which would help to prevent osteoporosis. Higher doses of oral estrogen, however, increase the level of HDL (the good cholesterol that helps to prevent heart disease). The patch did not.

As with oral estrogen, transdermal estrogen therapy will probably require that progestin, another hormone, be taken orally to help prevent the development of endometrial cancer in women who have not had a hysterectomy, the researchers say.

Patches of the Future

Not all drugs lend themselves to transdermal delivery. Some may irritate the skin, and the molecules of others may be too big to get through the skin. The drugs must be water-soluble and fat-soluble and effective in very low doses. For large doses such as you would need with antibiotics or aspirin, uncomfortably large patches would be required.

Scientists, however, are working on enhancers and special adhesives that will enable more drugs to be suitable for transdermal delivery. Here are some medications that may be available in patch form sometime in the future.

Narcotic analgesics. "This is one of the uses for the patch that may be the most important that will ever come," says Gordon Flynn, Ph.D., professor of pharmaceutics at the University of Michigan. "Potent analgesics can be narcotics. But we're not worrying about making addicts of people who are dying of cancer. No other analgesics will get to that deep-seated chronic pain that is almost enough to turn someone insane. It's badly managed now. The drugs we use are very short-acting and they're upsetting to the stomach. A tablet or a capsule doesn't last very long, so patients need to take another dose frequently. In the early part of the cycle, they don't have pain, but they quickly become sleepy. The body eliminates the drug, and they become uncomfortable again.

"A patch could probably reduce medical costs and make the family and patient happier. By the 1990s, certainly, this will be available. The good that will be done is incalculable."

Insulin. "Insulin molecules are normally too large to go through the skin. However, we have developed a special instrument that can deliver insulin and is so portable that it can be worn every day," says Yie W. Chien, Ph.D., chairman of Rutgers College of Pharmacy, Department of Pharmaceutics, and head of the Rutgers Controlled Drug Delivery Research Center. "This device uses a very acceptable level of electrical current, which will allow insulin to penetrate the skin without a needle. Tests are being done on a diabetic animal, and the results have been very encouraging. We hope to begin the clinical studies that will take a year or two. After that it must be approved by the FDA."

Contraceptives. "If all goes well with the clinical trials, a contraceptive patch should be available to the public in two to three years," says Dr. Chien. "A woman would apply one patch each week for a month in a continuing cycle. The patches would have varying amounts of medication, designed to replicate a woman's normal physiologic cycle. And the patch is so easy it will probably increase proper usage," says Dr. Chien.

Antihistamines. Twenty volunteers at the College of Pharmacy at North Dakota State University tested antihistamine patches to suppress allergy symptoms. The patches worked as well as antihistamine pills. Some people developed a mild itch around the patch site. The amount of drowsiness (a common side effect with antihistamines) was pretty much the same for the patches and pills. Further testing must be done to find the lowest, most effective dose and the length of time the patch is effective.

Nicotine. Like nicotine gum, this patch can help eliminate the craving for cigarettes. "Some people have said that the gum causes mouth ulceration and stomach upset and tastes really bad," says Frank Etscorn, Ph.D., psychology professor at New Mexico Tech in Socorro, and one of the developers of the nicotine patch. "We haven't found that nicotine irritates the skin.

"With the patch, smokers may be able to safely and gradually lower their dose and quit the habit without the harmful tars or carbon monoxide they get from smoking. Such a delivery system is being tested in England," where it may be on the market in the not-too-distant future, says Dr. Etscorn.

With this new generation of medications come new problems. Children love adhesive strips. Obviously, care must be taken in the storage and disposal of the patches. In one case, a patch was inadvertently transferred from an adult to a child who slept in his parents' bed. The child appeared noticeably sick all day, but the patch, which had stuck on his back, was not discovered until he was given his evening bath. So any missing patches should be accounted for.

The patches are more costly than pills, in some cases. But for people who forget to take their pills or who have severe side effects from oral medications, the patch may be a lifesaver.

CHAPTER 18
Ulcers: On the Brink of a Cure

Exciting new research may help duodenal ulcer patients finally find permanent relief—with a very familiar remedy.

For the millions of Americans who suffer from duodenal ulcer, the most common form of ulcer, doctors can offer little more than a good news/bad news prognosis. The good news: Conventional therapy—drugs that either reduce or neutralize acid or coat the stomach lining—can heal most ulcers in four to six weeks. The bad news: Healing is not curing.

"In an estimated 75 to 90 percent of cases, the ulcer recurs. In fact, roughly 10 to 20 percent of those who have surgery for duodenal ulcer still have some symptoms, and in 10 percent the ulcer returns. There's an old dictum in gastroenterology," says one researcher. " 'Once an ulcer, always an ulcer.' "

But new findings may change all that. Two Australian doctors have isolated bacteria that they think may be responsible for many if not all duodenal ulcers and chronic gastritis. Their theory is that relapse rates are high in ulcer cases because standard treatment never eradicates the ulcer's cause.

Most important, they believe that at the same time they may have found a cure that is simple, inexpensive and quick. It involves antibiotics and an over-the-counter medication that most Americans have probably used at some time for upset stomach or traveler's diarrhea.

In 1979, Robin Warren, a pathologist, and Barry Marshall, M.D., a gastroenterologist at the Royal Perth Hospital, discovered that an odd strain of bacteria was present in nearly all the test samples obtained from a group of patients with active chronic gastritis. Gastritis is a condition that frequently precedes or accompanies full-blown duodenal ulcer.

Over the next few years, Dr. Warren and Dr. Marshall tested hundreds of patients with gastritis and duodenal ulcer and in most found this spiral bacteria, which appeared to them to be a form of *campylobacter.* The most common *campylobacter* bacteria is known to cause diarrhea in humans. They named the new strain *Campylobacter pyloridis* because of its location in the stomach near the pylorus, the valve that holds food in the stomach.

At the same time, they began experimenting with a compound that had been shown to heal duodenal ulcer and, in fact, has a lower relapse rate than more conventional treatments. The substance is a compound of a heavy metal called bismuth, which had been used to treat syphilis and other bacterial infections before the discovery of penicillin in the 1940s. A very similar compound is the main ingredient of a common American over-the-counter remedy, Pepto-Bismol.

What Dr. Marshall and Dr. Warren found was that in a surprising number of cases, the bismuth compound worked. For many of the patients, not only did the bacteria disappear but so did their ulcers. In their most recent study, the researchers found that about 30 percent of ulcer patients who took the bismuth compound alone were clear of the bacteria, compared to none in the group given the usual ulcer treatment, cimetidine (Tagamet).

But the best clearance—75 percent—came in the group given the bismuth compound and an antibacterial drug similar to a prescription medication sold in the United States under the trade name Flagyl.

Of course, the real test for any ulcer treatment is the relapse rate. Reports Dr. Marshall, "When we did the relapse study, we found the relapse rate was proportional to the number of patients who still had the germ after treatment. The relapse rate was between 80 and 100 percent in all the Tagamet patients. It was between 50 and 70 percent in the patients who got the bismuth and placebo. But the relapse rate was only about 30 percent in the patients who got the bismuth and antibiotic."

The Tagamet patients were subsequently given the antibiotic and bismuth and, says Dr. Marshall, "they're all well. In fact, we have hardly had any patients requiring further treatment."

How It Works

How does *campylobacter* cause gastritis and duodenal ulcer in the first place? Dr. Marshall and his colleagues believe the bacteria, which can live in the acid environment of the stomach, either digests or in some way damages the mucous lining of the stomach. Without that protective lining, which he describes as "like plastic wrap," acid irritates and eventually eats a hole in the stomach, causing an ulcer.

The bacteria theory may explain why so many ulcers run in families. Scientists have long believed there was some genetic component to ulcers, though the exact connection has never been established. "We don't know how this bacterium is spread," says Dr. Marshall, "but there's some suggestion that it's through kissing, because husbands with duodenal ulcers often have wives who have gastritis. In fact, about half the wives of duodenal ulcer patients have gastritis."

More Ulcer Help from the Drugstore

While the Pepto-Bismol ulcer cure is still under investigation, there may be another alternative that's also as close as the pharmacy shelf.

Researchers have found that the regular daily use of the common antacid Maalox can prevent the relapse of duodenal ulcers.

In a multicenter study, researchers used a form of Maalox called Maalox TC, which has 2½ to 3 times the acid-buffering capacity of regular Maalox, on a group of duodenal ulcer patients.

Out of 173 patients with healed ulcers, only 25 percent had a recurrence within a year after taking three tablets every morning and night, according to one of the researchers, Chesley Hines, M.D., of the Ochsner Clinic in New Orleans. The greatest benefit was reaped by smokers in the study. "It's been shown clearly that ulcers recur more frequently in smokers, so it would make sense that a program to prevent recurrence would benefit smokers the most," explains Dr. Hines.

The researchers compared the Maalox TC to both cimetidine (Tagamet) and a harmless placebo (dummy pill) and, while the cimetidine users had only a slightly higher recurrence rate, there is less risk of side effects with the Maalox TC. (Oddly enough, there was one side effect that struck a few patients in all three groups, including those who were taking the nontherapeutic placebo: diarrhea. Dr. Hines has no explanation for why the placebo caused diarrhea, although it's a common side effect for most antacids.)

Maalox TC is readily available over the counter. Unlike the Pepto-Bismol/antibiotic treatment, though, it must be taken regularly.

Nevertheless, *Campylobacter pyloridis* does not appear to be highly infectious, though it's been estimated that as many as 40 percent of middle-aged Americans have it (compared to only 10 percent of young adults). Many of them, however, are symptomless.

One of the fortunate aspects of the Australian discovery—technically a rediscovery, since the bacterium was observed and promptly forgotten at least 40 years ago—is that the cure was not far behind. And it is an inexpensive cure. Conventional therapy, which includes indefinite maintenance, can cost roughly $1,000 or more over a period of five years, estimates Dr. Marshall. "And even then you still get a high relapse rate," he says.

Campylobacter pyloridis is very susceptible to the bismuth compound. Even if the antibiotic stops working, as it sometimes does, the bismuth continues to fight the bacteria, says Dr. Marshall. The germs don't seem to build up any immunity to it. And bismuth is easily and inexpensively available in Pepto-Bismol. "A two-week therapy of the bismuth compound and the antibiotic, which is really all that's usually needed, costs around $30," says the researcher. "And with this new therapy we're *curing* around 75 percent of the patients, and the treatment doesn't have to go on for months. That's because it's not just a treatment, it's a cure."

Another advantage is the lack of significant side effects, though Dr. Marshall cautions that none of the *campylobacter* studies, including his own, have been large enough or long enough to rule out possible side effects. He has now undertaken a clinical trial using the bismuth/antibiotic treatment on nonulcer dyspepsia, a related digestive disorder in which victims have gastritis without ulcer. "We want to see if we can prevent a relapse of nonulcer dyspepsia in exactly the same way as we prevent relapse of duodenal ulcer," he says.

Though other researchers have had some success with Pepto-Bismol alone, Dr. Marshall found that the bacteria tended to recolonize in many cases, so the one-two punch of bismuth and antibiotic appears to be necessary to eradicate the bug totally.

No Treatment Yet

Needless to say, the Australian findings have been causing a stir in the gastroenterological community since the first study appeared in the prestigious British journal *Lancet.*

But the Australian studies, while intriguing to the medical community, are still preliminary. Though the work is promising, Pepto-Bismol and antibiotics are unlikely to become the treatment of choice overnight. They represent a revolutionary treatment for ulcer, a condition which, up until this point, has been attacked from one direction: acid reduction.

"This is a fresh breeze, a new direction," says Frank Lanza, M.D., of Baylor College of Medicine in Houston, who did a study in which a two- to three-week dose of Pepto-Bismol alone healed and prevented the recurrence of gastritis in a small group of patients. "We are finally getting away from the 'acid is everything' thinking. We couldn't keep attacking this problem in the same old ways. We could heal ulcers, but the only way to prevent recurrence was to keep giving patients drugs indefinitely. Although ulcer drugs like cimetidine are relatively innocuous, they do have some systemic side effects."

The Australians have done more than simply stand by their work. In fact, Dr. Marshall was so convinced of the connection between this new bacterium and gastritis and ulcer that he swallowed a colony of *Campylobacter pyloridis* himself as a test, developed gastritis and cured it with a dose of bismuth and antibiotic.

These days, some of the big guns in gastroenterology are starting to pay attention, which could spell relief earlier than expected for ulcer and gastritis sufferers. "There are some very serious people involved in this research now," says Dr. Lanza.

CHAPTER 19

Fighting High Blood Pressure with Modern Medicines

An update on the best drugs available for hypertension.

Without a doubt, the greatest advance in the battle against hypertension has been the development of an array of effective drugs that lower blood pressure. These are all relatively new medications, introduced in the last 35 years. And even now, other new antihypertensive medications are being developed.

Before the 1950s, there was little that doctors could do to effectively treat primary hypertension. There was even less hope for patients with malignant hypertension—a form of the disease that progresses rapidly and, unless reversed, brings death within a few months. At the Cleveland Clinic, Irvine Page, M.D., widely acknowledged as the father of modern antihypertensive therapy, and his colleagues were undertaking their studies on the effects of renin, serotonin and other body chemicals that raise blood pressure. *Time* magazine, in its October 31, 1955, cover story on Dr. Page, quoted him as saying, "Hypertension is not a single disease. It may be almost as variable as the many different forms of cancer. Neither can it have a single cause. There are at least eight mechanisms in the body operating to maintain an even blood pressure, and these are all interrelated. The balance of one cannot be upset without upsetting the balance of the others."

But although Dr. Page was at the forefront in hypertension research and treatment, before the 1950s he still had little he could offer patients in the way of specific treatments. He used kidney extracts to treat malignant hypertension, with varying degrees of success. He also pioneered the use of hypothermia, or fever treatments, again with only moderate success.

For the more common forms of primary hypertension, Dr. Page and his colleagues could do little more than recommend "massive doses of moderation." To quote the same 1955 issue of *Time:* "First, they reassure the patient by explaining what they can do about his disease. Then they advise him to do what he can to avoid fatigue and excitement. He should spend ten hours in bed and take short naps, often. Every extra pound . . . means work for the heart, so reduce. Moderation is also prescribed in smoking and drinking, in exercise and sexual activity."

At that time, severe salt restriction also was used to treat high blood pressure, but again with only moderate success. At Duke University Medical Center, Walter Kempner, M.D., developed the rice diet that still bears his name. It cut salt consumption to 1⁄10 teaspoon a day, and it did lower high blood pressure in a large number of patients. This in itself was lifesaving in an era when there were no effective antihypertensive drugs. But for the less life-threatening forms of mild to moderate hypertension, the diet was so boring and restricted that most patients had difficulty adhering to it outside a hospital setting. Dr. Page noted that while the rice diet was certainly better than nothing, "a mere 25 percent of patients get their blood pressure down to near-normal levels" by following it, probably because most patients simply could not adhere to it on a long-term basis. Dr. Page supported salt restriction, but in the context of a more normal diet than the rice regimen.

The First Antihypertensive Agents

To realize just how significant antihypertensive drugs have become in the treatment of high blood pressure, one needs only to go back to 1944 and review the circumstances of President Roosevelt's death. As recalled by Edward Frohlich, M.D., a world authority on antihypertensive drugs who began his research career at the Cleveland Clinic and is now head of education, research and the hypertension section at the Ochsner Clinic, "FDR had severe hypertension, and the only means available then for his treatment was phenobarbital. Initially, there had been some concept that the brain was involved in the elevation of blood pressure, and phenobarbital was the only substance we had that reduced activity of the brain. Now we know that this serves only as a placebo." President Roosevelt died of hypertension at the relatively young age of 63.

In 1951, the outlook for patients with hypertension began to change dramatically with the administration of the first effective antihypertensive drug at the Cleveland Clinic. The patient was a 50-year-old soft drink manufacturer whose blood pressure was 230/146. He had an enlarged and failing heart and suffered from breathlessness, weakness and edema (swelling). Dr. Page and his colleagues had been studying hydralazine, a vasodilator drug, and they decided to administer it to this patient. (Vasodilators are a class of medications that relax the smooth muscles in the arteries.)

Hydralazine acts very quickly. Within 15 minutes after an intravenous injection of the drug, it begins to lower blood pressure. In a few hours the patient's blood pressure dropped, and over the next few months his other problems began to subside. Eventually, he was able to return to work and again lead a reasonably normal life, even though his heart remained enlarged.

Hydralazine is still used in treating high blood pressure, but it is no longer a first-choice drug. Its introduction at the Cleveland Clinic was quickly followed by the introduction of two other classes of drugs that lower blood pressure: hexamethonium and reserpine, a drug derived from the root of an Indian plant, rauwolfia.

Although the introduction of these drugs represented a major breakthrough in the treatment of hypertension, they were not without problems. Hydralazine can cause headaches and tachycardia (rapid heartbeat), and it is not recommended for patients with coronary artery disease or congestive heart failure. It also can cause gastrointestinal upsets, flushing, difficulty in breathing upon exertion, rashes and, in rare instances, nerve and blood problems. Hexamethonium and related drugs cause postural hypotension, which is a marked drop in blood pressure and fainting or light-headedness upon standing. This is an obvious problem for patients who are not bedridden, and the drugs have largely been replaced by other, more effective drugs with fewer side effects. Reserpine is still used but usually in combination with other drugs. Taken alone, reserpine is not potent enough to lower high blood pressure. The drug also has a number of potential side effects, including depression, lethargy, nightmares, nasal congestion, bradycardia (slow heartbeat) and diarrhea. It can also cause a buildup of sodium and body fluid.

The Diuretics

In 1958, chlorothiazide was introduced, and again the treatment of hypertension took a giant step forward. Chlorothiazide is the prototype of the thiazide diuretics—a group of drugs that lower blood pressure by increasing the kidney's excretion of sodium and water. These drugs are particularly useful for patients whose high blood pressure is related to increased blood volume and who have problems with accumulation of body fluid. But they seem to work in most patients with mild to moderate hypertension. In fact, studies at the Cleveland Clinic and elsewhere have found that two-thirds of all patients with mild to moderate hypertension can be adequately treated with a thiazide diuretic alone. In explaining why he prefers these drugs as the initial antihypertensive agents, one doctor says that they are generally well tolerated and that a single low dose of 12.5 milligrams a day is often sufficient. They are also less costly than most other antihypertensive drugs.

A low dose also minimizes the most common side effects of these drugs, which include metabolic problems (a rise in uric acid, blood sugar, cholesterol and triglycerides and a reduction in potassium) and sexual dysfunction in men. Since thiazides promote the excretion of potassium as well as sodium and chloride, their prolonged use may result in hypokalemia, a potentially dangerous deficiency of potassium. These problems usually can be avoided if the daily dosage of hydrochlorothiazide is less than 50 milligrams, according to one doctor. Even so, patients on thiazide diuretics should have their potassium levels measured regularly. Potassium loss may be increased by episodes of diarrhea or vomiting. Potassium is essential for the proper function of muscles, including the heart. If potassium levels fall too low, a potassium supplement may be prescribed.

Since 1958, a number of other potent diuretic drugs have been developed. All diuretics promote the excretion of sodium and fluid, but they have different sites of action. The loop diuretics, which include furosemide and ethacrynic acid, are so named because they work in the part of the kidney known as the loop of Henle. They are more potent than the thiazides and are usually reserved for patients whose blood pressure is not adequately lowered by the thiazides or who have impaired kidney function or a buildup of fluid in the lungs and heart. Loop diuretics also can deplete the body of potassium, even more rapidly than the thiazides. They also can cause a buildup of uric acid, which may result in attacks of gout.

Still another class of diuretics is the potassium-sparing agents: amiloride, spironolactone and triamterene. These drugs work in the exchange sites of the kidney tubules, enabling them to increase sodium excretion while sparing the potassium. Care must be taken, however, to prevent hyperkalemia, an excess of potassium, which may occur in patients with kidney failure. They are often prescribed along with a thiazide or a loop diuretic, which minimizes the potassium excretion and other problems and at the same time increases their effectiveness against edema. Spironolactone may cause gynecomastia, an abnormal breast enlargement in men. As with all diuretics, these drugs may cause sexual problems in men.

Since their introduction in the late 1950s and early 1960s, diuretics have been the mainstay antihypertensive drugs. Recently, however, their long-term safety has been questioned by several experts. These critics of diuretic therapy cite results from the long-term Multiple Risk Factor Intervention Trial (MRFIT), a study designed to determine the effects of reducing risk factors on deaths from heart attacks. When death rates among the various groups of MRFIT participants were compared, it was found that a subset of high-risk hypertensive men with abnormal resting electrocardiograms (EKGs) had a higher-than-expected death rate. The subset had been divided into two groups, one designated as special intervention (SI) and the other as usual care (UC). Both groups had received diuretics, but the special intervention group had been given higher dosages. One of the researchers notes that "many of these excess deaths were sudden and unexpected, suggesting arrhythmias, perhaps from diuretic-induced hypokalemia, although this has never been proved." He also stresses that among men who had abnormal exercise EKGs, the mortality rate was lower in the SI group than the UC subset. Also, other studies involving long-term users of diuretics have failed to document an increased risk of death. In fact, the researcher stresses that all of the studies that have found a reduction in cardiovascular illness and deaths have used a diuretic as the first-choice drug, and only MRFIT has raised a question about their safety. "All drugs carry some risk, but I have no doubt that there is more risk involved in untreated hypertension than there is in treating it with diuretics," he says.

Beta-Adrenergic Blockers

These drugs, commonly referred to as beta-blockers, were first introduced in the United States about 20 years ago for the treatment of angina. Propranolol was the first of the beta-blockers to be approved by the U.S. Food and Drug Administration; since then, a half dozen others have been introduced.

Beta-blockers act by inhibiting responses of the beta

receptors in the autonomic nervous system. This has numerous effects, particularly upon the heart. Propranolol, which is considered the prototype beta-blocker, reduces the oxygen demand of the heart muscle, which slows the heart rate and reduces the amount of blood pumped out. It was first used to treat angina, the chest pains that result when the heart muscle is not getting enough blood. It was soon discovered that the drug also lowered blood pressure.

About half of all patients with mild hypertension can be treated with beta-blockers alone. These drugs are particularly useful for patients who have coronary artery disease and episodes of angina or cardiac arrhythmias in addition to high blood pressure. Studies have shown that patients given a beta-blocker following a heart attack are less likely to suffer a subsequent heart attack or sudden death. Since they do not affect uric acid levels, they are useful for hypertensive patients who also suffer from gout. These drugs should not be taken by patients with congestive heart failure and should be used along with a diuretic by patients with edema. They are contraindicated for patients with bradycardia, asthma or chronic lung disease, since they may worsen these conditions. Beta-blockers tend to increase blood cholesterol and triglycerides and to lower the protective HDL cholesterol. But these changes usually are not enough to contraindicate their use in patients who have coronary disease, since their protective effect probably exceeds the adverse effect of a modest rise in cholesterol.

Most patients tolerate beta-blockers well. About 5 percent of patients complain of unusual tiredness or lethargy while taking beta-blockers. Some men experience impotence or loss of sexual desire. Other, less common, adverse reactions include depression, mood changes, nightmares or vivid dreams, itching or other skin irritations, gastrointestinal upsets and respiratory problems.

Individual people may react differently to different beta-blockers. For example, if one causes impotence or some other undesirable side effect, the problem may be solved by lowering the dosage or switching to another beta-blocker.

Care must be taken not to abruptly stop a beta-blocker, since this may result in a worsening of angina or even precipitate a heart attack. When going off a beta-blocker, the dosage should gradually be decreased over a one- to two-week period, with special attention paid to any symptoms that may indicate a worsening heart problem.

Alpha-Adrenergic Blockers

Like beta-blockers, these drugs also work through the autonomic nervous system by blocking the alpha receptors. They lower blood pressure by dilating the arterioles (tiny blood vessels) and are generally used in combination with other antihypertensive drugs. Alpha-blockers also interfere with the action of stress hormones.

Prazosin is the major drug in this category; it is less likely to cause tachycardia than other alpha-blockers. But it can cause postural hypotension, especially after the first dose. Patients who are just beginning treatment with prazosin should be careful about standing suddenly, since this may produce a sudden drop in blood pressure and dizziness or fainting. Prazosin is particularly useful for patients who have congestive heart failure or pheochromocytoma, a type of tumor that produces the hormones epinephrine and norepinephrine.

Centrally Acting Drugs

These drugs lower blood pressure by suppressing the sympathetic nervous system, thereby reducing heart rate, the heart's output of blood and the resistance of the peripheral blood vessels. Drugs in this category include methyldopa, clonidine and guanabenz. They are prescribed with a diuretic and are reserved for patients whose blood pressure is not sufficiently lowered with a diuretic alone or by a diuretic and a beta-blocker.

Drowsiness, dryness of the mouth and constipation are the most common adverse reactions. Sometimes dizziness or postural hypotension occurs, usually at the beginning of treatment. Some patients, especially those in jobs that demand mental sharpness, also complain about a reduction in their ability to think clearly. Care must be taken not to stop these drugs abruptly; this can cause serious rebound hypertension and a hypertensive crisis due to the sudden release of norepinephrine, a stress hormone.

Peripheral Adrenergic Antagonists

These drugs lower blood pressure by interfering with the release of norepinephrine from sympathetic nerve endings in response to a stimulus. Reserpine is one of the older antihypertensive agents. Other drugs in this category include guanadrel and guanethidine.

Reserpine is sometimes used alone to treat mild or moderate hypertension, but more often the drug is used along with a thiazide diuretic for patients whose blood pressure is not controlled with a diuretic alone. Guanethidine is a more potent antihypertensive drug and is usually prescribed for patients with severe hypertension that is not controlled by other drug regimens. Its major side effect is postural hypotension. Another drug, guanadrel, is not as potent as guanethidine, but it has similar (though less frequent and less severe) side effects. It is used in treating milder hypertension, usually with a diuretic. Sodium retention and water retention may occur with drugs in this category if they are not given along with a diuretic. Patients taking reserpine may encounter central nervous system problems, such as lethargy, nightmares and mental depression; the drug should not be taken by patients who have suffered from depression, and it should be discontinued if symptoms of depression occur.

Vasodilators

These are drugs that dilate or expand the blood vessels, thereby allowing blood to flow through them with less resistance. Hydralazine, the oldest antihypertensive agent, is a vasodilator; other drugs in this category include diazoxide, minoxidil and nitroprusside. As noted earlier, these drugs have a number of side effects, but they are useful when combined in small doses with other antihypertensive agents to lower blood pressure that is resistant to other treatments. They are also useful in hypertensive emergencies because they act quickly with a dramatic lowering of blood pressure. Minoxidil is one of the most potent of all antihypertensive drugs, but it causes excessive growth of facial and body hair (hirsutism).

Converting Enzyme Inhibitors

These are among the newest antihypertensive drugs. They lower blood pressure by blocking the enzyme that converts angiotensin I to angiotensin II, one of the body's most potent chemicals that increase blood pressure. Angiotensin is produced in response to the release of renin from the kidney; therefore, these drugs are particularly useful in treating hypertensive patients whose high blood pressure is related to excessive renin activity. Drugs in this category are captopril and enalapril. They are usually prescribed with a diuretic, which increases their effectiveness.

Special care must be taken in giving these drugs to people with kidney disease; kidney failure has occurred in some patients with preexisting loss of kidney function. Other adverse reactions include blood disorders, rashes, hypotension and a reversible loss of taste.

Calcium Channel Blockers

These also are new drugs and are used mostly for angina, particularly the type that is caused by a spasm of a coronary artery and occurs while a patient is at rest. Calcium channel blockers interfere with the action of calcium on the artery muscles, resulting in a dilation of the blood vessels and a drop in blood pressure. Drugs in this category include verapamil, diltiazem and nifedipine. They are usually prescribed with a diuretic, and their use with a beta-blocker is generally avoided. Calcium channel blockers are not for patients who have heart block or other disturbances in their cardiac electrical system. Adverse reactions with calcium channel blockers include headaches, dizziness, palpitations, gastrointestinal disturbances, rashes and swelling of the lower legs.

Special Considerations

When beginning antihypertensive therapy, a patient should see his or her physician frequently, sometimes every week or two. This allows a doctor to monitor the effectiveness of the drugs and to adjust dosages, check on adverse reactions and find out if there are any other problems. Often, patients are reluctant to bring up certain side effects, or they think they must suffer in order for the drugs to work. Still others drop out of treatment, especially if the drugs make them feel sicker than before they started therapy. In reality, most side effects can be controlled or minimized, either by adjusting the dosage or by switching drugs. Others are temporary and will cease once the body becomes adjusted to the drug.

PART IV: MEDICAL TESTS AND YOUR HEALTH

CHAPTER 20
Which Test Spots Allergies Best?

A Prevention *writer gives a first-person account of the tests and a rating for each.*

Whenever allergists get together, sooner or later the talk turns to testing. Some will vigorously defend the traditional skin-prick method, while others will endorse tests that use the patient's blood instead.

This time I went beyond talking to the experts and got the inside story. An allergy sufferer since birth, I actually took all the tests I'll be discussing.

I was skin-tested on my back and arms. I gave blood that was analyzed in one office via the MAST system, sent to Texas for a FAST test and shipped to Johns Hopkins University School of Medicine for RAST testing. There were intradermal tests to double-check skin-test results.

Over $1,000 was spent to come to the conclusion that the single most important indicator of allergy problems is also the least expensive and causes absolutely no discomfort. No needles enter your veins and no pins prick your skin, yet it provides your allergist with the information that's necessary to narrow the cause of your symptoms down to a few possibilities.

Talk May Be Cheap, But It's Sure Accurate

"Any test you run is only as good as the medical history you've taken to help you interpret these results," explains Mark P. Shampain, M.D., the Pennsylvania allergist who performed the tests.

"A good allergist," says Dr. Shampain, "sits down with the patient and asks a lot of questions before any testing takes place—questions about symptoms, possible triggers, food-related problems, medical history, medications and allergies in the family."

Before Dr. Shampain speaks with a patient, he has the patient fill out a detailed four-page questionnaire that asks more questions than the IRS. You not only have to identify your problems, you also must try to remember what age you were when they started, how often they bother you and which months are the worst.

You're asked about pets, exposure to smokers at home or work, where you've lived over the years, the construction of those residences and the contents of your pillows, as well as what type of heating you have, what your carpets are made of and what kind of work you do.

Filling in the blanks means calling family members to ask which ancestors had allergies. Pillows, mattresses and rugs have to be checked to see what they're made of or stuffed with. Hardest of all can be trying to remember in June what your symptoms were like in January!

But even incomplete and peppered with "best guesses," a filled-in form and an interview can convey as much information as any test that will later be run.

The Old Skin Game

"The skin-prick test is one of the most accurate diagnostic tests known to man," says Charles H. Banov, M.D., past president of the American College of Allergists.

"You're testing the actual allergic individual with an extract of the specific substance that is suspected of causing the problems. And the doctor interprets the results of that test while actually looking at the patient. You can see the reactions.

"A good allergist starts by taking a careful history and then running skin tests to confirm his suspicions. If those tests are indecisive, then it makes sense to draw blood and conpare the results—but those cases are one in a thousand. I have as busy an allergy practice as anyone, and I only order two or three allergy blood tests a year."

Writer on the Table

In the first week's skin tests, a total of 47 "inhalant" substances were tested. Dr. Shampain uses a system where a kind of scrub brush holding ten little pins, each coated with a different allergen, is pressed into your back. This isn't as tedious as endless single pricks.

Histamine, which everyone—allergies or not—will react to, is also tested as a control. This makes sure that "no results" really means "no allergies" and not that the patient had taken antihistamines or that some other factor was interfering with the tests.

After 15 minutes, the area where six different grasses were tested had merged into one large, itchy welt. There were also strong reactions to weeds, trees, cats, dogs, feathers and tobacco—and a dust mite reaction that felt like a Texas mosquito bite.

To gauge the test results, small rulers are used to measure the diameter of the "wheals" that flare up. The redness of the area is also assigned a relative number. (The after-effects of the test are fairly easy to control—an antihistamine and some anesthetic ointment, such as Lidex, end the itch very quickly.)

The raised wheals corresponding to the grasses, pets and mites lingered for days, but surprisingly, without itching or discomfort. Fresh mosquito bites are a lot worse.

The reactions to foods were much less pronounced, and Dr. Shampain was not surprised. "You rarely see as big a reaction with foods," he explained.

Since there was a history of severe reaction to shrimp and other seafood, Dr. Shampain tested for these separately. He used my arm, "so we can throw a tourniquet around it if you start to go into anaphylaxis."

Luckily, the shellfish reactions were as mild as the rest. But Dr. Shampain cautions that precautions should be taken to test carefully whenever there is a history of severe reactions.

He Got under My Skin

Curious about the lack of reactions to various molds tested the first week, Dr. Shampain used the other arm for a stronger form of skin testing—intradermal.

In skin-prick testing, a tiny break in the top layer of skin allows the smallest possible amount of the substance on the pin to come into contact with the body's cells. In intradermal testing, a larger amount of the substance is actually injected just under the skin. This type of test should never be done before prick testing, warn both Dr. Banov and Dr. Shampain, since the chance of a serious reaction is much stronger. (The molds still tested negative.)

The cat, dog, tobacco and dust mite reactions all corresponded well with my actual symptoms, but the strong reaction to grass and trees did not. Although this was the worst grass pollen season in decades, I had few outdoor symptoms. (Childhood reactions were another story—when neighbors mowed their lawn, I went to the emergency room.)

The skin tests were a real bargain: 35 substances cost only $78.75. That's less than half of what the cheapest blood tests cost.

MAST, FAST and RAST: The Blood Brothers

Over a period of weeks, blood was drawn for the three most common blood tests.

Dr. Shampain has a complete MAST system in his office that processes the blood and prints out the results. The FAST testing was supervised by allergist Lyndon Mansfield, M.D., and the RAST test was run by the allergy lab at

Johns Hopkins University School of Medicine in Baltimore.

MAST. The MAST system gives a digital readout for each substance tested that represents the strength of the

MAST, FAST and RAST— What's behind the Initials?

"All of these blood tests are based on the same 'sandwich' principle," explains Frederick Rommel, Ph.D., director of the DACI reference lab in the Allergy and Clinical Immunology Division of Johns Hopkins University School of Medicine in Baltimore.

In each test, a single allergy-causing substance—let's use ragweed as an example—is coated on a thread (MAST), coated on a plastic surface (FAST) or chemically bonded to paper (RAST) and exposed to the person's blood. Any of the IgE factor in that blood sensitive to ragweed will bind to it and become firmly attached.

Meanwhile, a substance called anti-IgE, which locks onto human IgE like the right piece of a jigsaw puzzle, is combined with either an enzyme (MAST and FAST) or radioactive iodine (RAST). This "activated" anti-IgE is then added to the ragweed sample that's still got the IgE from your blood firmly attached.

The anti-IgE locks onto the human IgE and holds tight. If your blood has a lot of IgE against ragweed, then a lot of anti-IgE will also hook up with it, making the completed "sandwich."

Still attached to that anti-IgE is either the specialized enzyme or the radioactive iodine. These elements are what each test really measures. It's complicated, but all you really have to remember is that the

allergic reaction. These numbers, like skin tests, are graded from 0 (no reaction) to 4 (strong reaction). As with the skin tests, my MAST numbers were high for grasses, trees, dust, mites and pets, and low for the molds.

more IgE in your blood against ragweed, the more radioactive iodine or enzyme "marker" will also wind up stuck to the ragweed sample.

MAST. A product of the 1980s, MAST modifies the FAST technique by testing 35 samples at once in a single module, with little individual chambers for each substance to be tested. You can actually see the fluorescence, recorded on a little strip on black and white Polaroid film that's supplied with the test results.

FAST. Developed in the 1970s, this system uses an enzyme like the ones that tenderize meat and digest our food. But when this enzyme eats, fluorescent light—like that of a firefly—is a by-product. The more IgE that sticks to the ragweed, the brighter the light that results.

RAST. Developed in the late 1960s, this is the original allergy blood test. Radioactive iodine-125 is bonded to the anti-IgE, and a counter (that functions like a Geiger counter) measures the gamma radiation from the iodine. The higher the count, the more IgE you have against ragweed, and, theoretically, the stronger your allergy to it.

Dr. Rommel points out that the costs for these tests will vary widely, depending on the lab. Their tests are expensive, he says, because they run each one twice with a negative or positive control. If the two results are different, it shows that something went wrong. Dr. Rommel frowns on tests that don't double-check themselves. "They're a real disservice to patients," he says.

But the MAST test claimed many more reactions to foods than did the skin tests. Both had shown a response to wheat, corn, soybeans and peanuts, but the MAST also found reactions to milk, pork, almonds, oats, rye and potatoes, plus a very strong reaction to rice.

The MAST results also provide a reading on the total IgE level of the blood. IgE is an antibody that is present in increased levels in people with allergies and thus is a good indicator of a person's allergic potential. My total IgE was in the "High to Very High" range—3.46 when the standard range is from 0.0 to 4.0.

"Less than 5 percent of the blood tests I've ever seen have come back this positive," explained Dr. Shampain, adding that "most people just don't get usable results." He says, "Skin tests are another story. They yield useful information better than 90 percent of the time."

The MAST test cost $200 for 35 substances.

FAST. FAST also indicated a reaction to grasses, but a much smaller reaction than the other tests. The FAST results were the highest for the "real" allergy triggers: house dust (a mix that includes mites), dog and cat all showed very strong reactions.

Most of the foods that MAST had shown reactions to tested negative. FAST instead found reactions to barley, shrimp, tomato and tuna. All the tests (except RAST, which was borderline negative) agreed on a high number for tomato, which causes an itchy mouth and other symptoms when I eat them raw.

Although only FAST showed a reaction, shrimp and tuna are considered deadly (due to old reactions), and I've avoided them for years.

The FAST price was $210 for 35 tests.

RAST. The RAST tests were run by Frederick Rommel, Ph.D., director of the DACI reference laboratory at Johns Hopkins University School of Medicine.

The most exceptional finding in the RAST results was a milk reading that was quite high. It was no surprise to Dr. Rommel, who says that "it's not uncommon to have positive readings for milk without any symptoms."

The RAST also picked up very high readings on many grasses but was lower for trees. House dust, cat, dog and two different species of dust mite all came up medium to high positive. Again, molds tested negative.

The RAST tests performed at Johns Hopkins don't come back in the standardized 0 to 4 range (although RAST tests

When Blood Tests Are Better

Here are some situations in which blood tests are the better method of testing for allergies.

- People with eczema tend to have underreactive skin that may not show results of skin tests very well. Other chronic skin conditions can also pose a problem.
- A small percentage of the population has needle phobia, and the thought of enduring dozens of pinpricks is their worst nightmare come true.
- Recent or chronic antihistamine use can prevent release of the histamine that skin tests depend on. Five days of abstinence cover most varieties, but some foreign drugs disrupt test results for months.
- Tricyclic antidepressants, like Elavil, have an antihistamine effect. Be sure that your allergist knows about all the medications you're taking. (Drugs don't affect blood tests.)
- If you use a pencil or other object to stroke the skin of someone with an allergic condition known as dermographism, you'll almost always raise a welt. Skin test results all look the same on these folks.
- Infants and fearful children will often tolerate the drawing of blood better than skin testing, which can be frightening and uncomfortable for the very young and highly allergic.

performed by other labs do), so it's difficult to compare numbers exactly, but the total IgE reading was very easy to interpret. The test's normal range is between 5 and 472 nanograms per milliliter (ng./ml.). My number was 1,943 ng./ml. "Elevated," was how Dr. Rommel put it, and this agreed nicely with the high MAST reading.

The RAST price was $490 for 35 tests at Johns Hopkins, but most labs would charge between $210 and $420.

Bad Blood?

"Blood tests for allergies aren't new," explains Dr. Banov. "They've been around since the 1960s. They're just being marketed very aggressively now. They're certainly no more accurate than skin tests, and they're much more expensive. Blood tests can also be plagued by false positives, indicating allergies that don't really exist, particularly if they're not interpreted in light of a patient's allergic history.

"One reason they're being pushed is that they're easy for the doctor—almost anyone can draw blood, and you don't have to keep a supply of fresh allergy extracts and trained personnel on hand as with skin tests."

Dr. Shampain has occasion to use the MAST system in his office only once or twice a month and feels that the other blood tests are "no better or worse."

"The problem with blood tests," explains Dr. Rommel, "is that the real allergic reaction takes place in the body when Mast cells are triggered by the substance that the person is allergic to." These are located in the skin and other organs of the body, *not* in the blood. The IgE factor in the blood is really just a "spillover" of the IgE that is not attached to these Mast cells.

"Skin tests are more accurate because you're testing the part of the body in which the allergic reaction actually occurs," he says.

For information about a new blood test that is reported to be inexpensive and highly accurate, see chapter 22, More Good News about Medical Tests.

CHAPTER 21

How to Check Out Your Cholesterol

When should you have it checked? What does it cost? And what do the numbers mean?

How do I know if I have it?

If "it" is poison ivy, a broken leg or incontinence, that's a question you probably won't need to ask. At the very least, you'll know that something is very wrong—enough to propel you to the doctor, if necessary.

But heart disease is different. Too much cholesterol in your blood works insidiously over decades, depositing layers of plaque that narrow arteries, slowing blood flow to a trickle and ending in a heart attack that could be fatal. All this without so much as a hint of trouble beforehand, in many cases.

That's why having your cholesterol level checked is so important. It's like taking a peek inside your arteries, like a sneak preview that gives you the chance to avoid a bad movie. And you can. Doctors have found that reducing a high cholesterol level reduces the risk of heart attack.

So how do you go about checking out your cholesterol? The best place to start is at your doctor's office. The next time you're there, simply ask to have your cholesterol tested. Or call to make an appointment to have it done.

It's best to do it at a time in your life when your diet is not changing a lot and you're not gaining or losing weight—what's called a steady state. "People say, 'Oh, I'm gonna get my cholesterol measured' and start changing their diet to the way they think they should eat," says John W. Farquhar, M.D., director of the Stanford Center for Research in Disease Prevention at Stanford University. "It's better to see what it is on your usual diet, then if you want to experiment, you can change and see what happens."

The test consists of having a small tube of blood drawn from your arm—about 10 cc, or ⅓ ounce—not exactly the

Cholesterol at Your Fingertips

There's a new technology afoot that could put cholesterol measurement at your fingertips.

It's called the finger-stick method, and its name describes the technique pretty well. A lancet is used to prick a fingertip, and a drop of blood is all the machine needs to perform the test.

"The finger-stick procedure promises to revolutionize the whole area of detection of elevated blood cholesterol," says Michael White, associate director for prevention, education and control for the National Heart, Lung and Blood Institute. "It provides an almost instant analysis."

The machines will probably be in most doctors' offices and will give them the ability to take an analysis and counsel patients on the spot. "The way it is now, doctors lose a lot of time between when the test is taken and when the patient comes back in—if they can get them back in at all," says White.

But the machines can save money as well as time. It's estimated that a cholesterol measurement by the finger-stick method will cost under $5.

"Several of the machines have already been approved by the Food and Drug Administration," says White. "They're being used in some mass screenings, but we feel they still need to be evaluated and improved before they'll be considered a very reliable tool. There's a general optimism, though, that that will take place in the near future—within the next year or two."

stuff horror films are made of. It's not usually painful, either. The blood can be drawn right in the doctor's office, although some physicians may send you to a laboratory to have it done.

If you're testing only for total cholesterol, the blood can be drawn on the spot. But if your doctor decides to test for triglycerides as well, you'll be instructed to fast before having the test. That means nothing to eat after dinner (about 6:00 P.M.) the night before the test. No chips during your favorite TV show. No ice cream during the 11 o'clock news. No real hardship. Schedule the test for first thing the following morning, and your fast will be over in short order.

Once the sample reaches the lab, a technician spins the tube of blood in a centrifuge to separate the cells from the serum. The cells end up in the bottom of the tube, with the serum on top, kind of like sediment resting at the bottom of a lake. A small sample of the serum is removed and a machine does the actual test. Depending on how busy the lab is, your doctor could have the results the next day.

What It All Means

The first thing to know about your cholesterol measurement is that you should take it with a grain of salt. "It's best not to think of it as a magical number that really is your number," says Dr. Farquhar. For one thing, your cholesterol level varies. "People know that there's variability in body weight, they know blood pressure bounces around, and they need to be told that cholesterol bounces around, too."

There's also variability at the laboratory. "Some of the variation is technical. There are different methods for measuring total cholesterol that give slightly different results," says John C. LaRosa, M.D., director of the Lipid Research Clinic at George Washington University School of Medicine and Health Sciences. "And there's probably some variation within laboratories, too." For those reasons, and because there can be an occasional fluke, Dr. LaRosa recommends that you have at least two cholesterol measurements done within two weeks. Dr. Farquhar recommends having it done three times and taking the average.

What's a safe cholesterol level? A panel of experts met in 1984 to decide that question, among others. That "consensus development panel," set up by the National Institutes of Health, issued a chart listing the risks of various cholesterol levels in people of various ages. It's so detailed that it's a little unwieldy. But it's probably safe to generalize that a cholesterol measurement over 200 milligrams per deciliter may be cause for concern. "Ideally, it should be 180 or below," says Dr. Farquhar.

Another question you might have is whether to have your levels of triglycerides and HDL cholesterol (high-density lipoprotein—the protective kind) checked while you're at it. There's no definitive answer yet, but that aspect of cholesterol testing is being considered as part of the work of an expert panel on detection, evaluation and treatment of high blood cholesterol. In the meantime, most doctors recommend using total cholesterol as a screening test, then checking further if the level is elevated.

"You're not going to get agreement on whether all of the tests ought to be done on everyone," says Dr. LaRosa. "But there's reasonable agreement that a total cholesterol point somewhere around 200 ought to be a trigger for separating people who probably don't need any more attention (provided there is no family history of heart disease) and people who need a triglyceride and HDL test. If there is a family history of heart disease, you probably ought to measure triglyceride and HDL anyway." Some doctors measure triglycerides and/or HDL cholesterol as a matter of course.

Hold the HDL?

One argument for holding off on HDL testing is that it has even more problems with accuracy than the total cholesterol test. In addition, it adds considerable expense. While a measurement of total cholesterol averages about $25, a full "cardiovascular profile" may cost $60 or more. (Check with your insurer about coverage.)

If you do have your HDL tested, the lab can then also calculate the level of LDL cholesterol (low-density lipoprotein—the dangerous kind). Basically, the more HDL, the better, and the less LDL, the better. An HDL below 40 or 50 is cause for concern; so is an LDL over 160.

But it's not cut and dried. Various genetic and environmental factors can influence these levels. Here's where the interpretation of the results gets pretty complicated—a good argument for doing all of this through your doctor.

Some doctors rely on the ratio between total cholesterol and HDL as an indication of risk. (The ratio is attained by dividing the total cholesterol number by the HDL number.) The lower the ratio, the better—that means that there's more HDL compared to LDL. A ratio below 3.5 would be considered ideal, a ratio of 4.0 to 5.0, about average risk. But there are situations where the ratio method doesn't work. One of those situations is when the total cholesterol level is in the upper 200s. If a person has a total cholesterol of 280, for example, and an HDL of 80, his ratio would be 3.5, which sounds pretty good, right? "I'd still worry about that person," says Dr. LaRosa. "The HDL is high, but the LDL is also very high. I'm not too reassured by high HDL in the presence of high LDL." Dr. Farquhar agrees, "If the LDL is high, I want to see it down. I don't want to trust the protection of HDL."

The first step in lowering a high cholesterol level is a change in diet. "Regardless of your cholesterol level, you should change your diet toward the prudent diet," says Dr. Farquhar. "If the test indicates moderate or high risk, you should start pursuing it more vigorously."

Dr. LaRosa agrees. "Everybody should be tried on a diet first," he says. "Most doctors would agree that the American Heart Association [AHA] diet is appropriate. It's actually a series of diets that starts by lowering cholesterol and saturated-fat content and increasingly lowering those components more and more as the 'phase' of the diet is increased." (Your local AHA can provide you with the details.)

Time to Change

Just don't expect immediate changes. "It takes time to get your mind made up, learn new habits of eating, change your palate preference around, get used to it, practice it and feel comfortable with it," says Dr. Farquhar. "Let's say that takes you two to three months. Once you've made the change, it takes only a week to ten days on that particular diet to affect your cholesterol level. Then you can go back and have your cholesterol checked two or three more times. If it hasn't gone down enough, then go into a more advanced nutritional-change program. Try that for three months. See if it works. If it still doesn't work, consider medications under your doctor's careful guidance."

If your doctor advises exercise and weight loss, you'll need even more patience. Those can take even longer to accomplish than changing the nature of your diet. "After you reach the weight you think you'll be able to maintain, stay there for a couple of weeks and get into a steady state before you get your cholesterol done again," says Dr. Farquhar.

If your cholesterol level is normal, keeping track of it is a much simpler affair. "Assuming that your cholesterol level is normal, the AHA has somewhat arbitrarily decided on checking it once every five years," says Dr. LaRosa. "But that's assuming that there's no major change in health, weight, diet or exercise patterns." If you're very concerned, you may want to have it checked every year.

The age at which to begin testing is another subject of intense debate. "I think all adults should have a cholesterol measurement done," says Dr. LaRosa. "Whether or not to screen all children is still debatable. Children with a strong family history of coronary disease should be tested. And I think it's very practical to say that children who go to a pediatrician for any reason should have a cholesterol test. But most people agree that in children under the age of two, it's not worth being concerned about."

CHAPTER 22

More Good News about Medical Tests

A review of some of the latest devices and ideas that could save your health.

Scientists are working overtime to perfect technology that can detect disease. Here's a sampling of their most recent, most promising efforts.

Gauge Your Kidney-Stone Risk with a New Home Test Kit

If you suffer from chronic kidney stones, a new medical test kit for use at home can help your physician diagnose the cause of stone formation—and let you know whether you're at risk of forming new stones.

Developed by researchers at the University of Texas Health Science Center in Dallas, the StoneRisk Patient Profile kits include material for urine sampling as well as a data card and mailing box so you can send samples directly to a central laboratory for analysis.

Your physician will receive computerized graph results of the samples, which make it easier to detect increased level of citrate—a substance that normally prevents kidney stones from forming—as well as other problems that could contribute to stone formation. Test results can also tell your physician which type of stones you're most likely to develop.

The StoneRisk Patient Profile test kit costs $250 and must be dispensed by a physician. For a product brochure, contact Mission Pharmaceutical Company, P.O. Box 1676, San Antonio, TX 78296 (800-531-3333; in Texas: 800-292-

7364). Your doctor can order a kit directly from the company.

Lung-Cancer Self-Test

By the time lung cancer shows up on an x-ray, it's usually too late. But a new test can show smokers precancerous changes in their lungs—while there may still be time for them to cure themselves by quitting. The test is a refinement of the sputum cytology test developed back in 1943 by George Papanicolaou, M.D., inventor of the Pap smear test that has saved countless women from death by early detection of cervical cancer.

The sputum test, called Novacyte, may help millions of smokers by showing lung-cell changes that could lead to or indicate cancer far earlier than x-rays can. Perhaps it may even goad some smokers into quitting.

The test is now available by prescription. You take it home and mail off a sputum specimen. The results are sent to your doctor for interpretation. The test manufacturer, Xsirius Medical, handles the analysis and informs your doctor of the results. They can also put you in touch with a doctor if you don't have one, provided you're over 40 and a smoker with a chronic cough.

At $90, the test may seem expensive, but think of the money you'll save when it convinces you to stop smoking. For more information, contact Xsirius Medical, Inc., 27520 Hawthorne Blvd., Suite 260, Rolling Hills Estates, CA 90274 (213-377-0848).

A New Kind of Allergy Test That Spares Your Skin

"To skin test—or not to skin test?" That's the question posed by many an allergic Hamlet. "Whether it is nobler to suffer the pinpricks of outrageous skin testing—or just give a tube of blood?"

Unfortunately, for those who want reliable results, there hasn't been much real choice. Although they can be uncomfortable and annoying, skin tests generally have been considered more reliable and less expensive than the various types of allergy blood testing available.

But not anymore. Researchers from the Emory University School of Medicine in Atlanta, Georgia, have developed a new, inexpensive blood test that seems to be highly accurate.

All they have to do is take some of your blood, incubate it with an extract of such well-known causes of allergy attack as dust, animal hair or pollen, and then measure the amount of histamine that your blood releases. That's it—none of the complicated mixing and bonding that make today's standard blood tests so time-consuming and expensive.

Using this new system, the researchers tested 150 people with allergies. Skin tests and detailed questioning were used to figure out the people's actual allergies. Then their blood was tested for comparison.

The results of this study showed a 90 to 100 percent agreement between the histamine release and skin testing. The popular RAST blood test has an overall accuracy rate of only about 70 percent.

The development of an inexpensive and accurate blood test is something that allergists and patients alike have long been hoping for. The authors of the report on this new test point out that it also avoids the possibility of extremely allergic individuals having a reaction during skin testing.

Picture Cervical Cancer Eliminated

A new screening technique that is reliable and inexpensive may help make cervical cancer a disease of the past. It's called cervicography, and it consists of taking a picture of the cervix by means of a special photographic instrument called a cerviscope. The slide, or cervigram, can later be magnified on a screen for experts in cervical cancer to read, much like the reading of an x-ray.

In a recent study of over 3,000 women between the ages of 18 and 50, this new diagnostic tool was found to be 4.5 times more sensitive in detecting precancerous changes than the Pap test.

Another study showed false-negative rates (when cancer is present but not detected) for cervicography to be 20 percent, compared to 64 percent for the Pap test.

"Because of the high false-negative rate, the Pap smear did not eliminate all cervical cancer as it was intended to," says Adolph Stafl, M.D., Ph.D., professor of gynecology and obstetrics at the Medical College of Wisconsin, who invented the cerviscope. "By combining the two techniques, we might be able to eliminate all cervical cancer," he says.

Dr. Stafl still recommends that a Pap smear be done every year. "The cervigram will be necessary only a few times in a woman's lifetime," he says. "A woman is at highest risk for precancerous cells developing at puberty and early adolescence and with her first pregnancy. This is when a cervigram is helpful to see if the cells are changing and determine if the woman is at risk for cervical cancer." If precancerous lesions are found, treatment such as cauterization or freezing of the abnormal tissue can be done to reduce the risk of developing cancer.

In any case, the cervigram can be kept as a permanent photographic record that can be used for comparison if the need arises at some point in the future.

Cervicography is now being used in over 200 locations in the United States. It is also being used in Europe, China and Australia. Because the photographic equipment is relatively inexpensive, Dr. Stafl believes it will be affordable for most examining rooms.

Smell Detection

"Scratch and sniff" has found a new use—in a smell-disorder test. The new test is fast and easy to do and may become the medical standard. It's being used in about 700 clinics by neurologists and otolaryngologists to screen patients for loss of smell, which can be a symptom of more than 30 disorders, including asthma, multiple sclerosis and Parkinson's disease.

Developed by Richard L. Doty, Ph.D., director of the University of Pennsylvania Clinical Smell and Taste Research Center, the new test replaces the messy and less accurate sniff bottles used until now.

Faster Temperature Taking

New urinary thermometers may streamline temperature taking. Doctors have known for more than 50 years that the temperature of urine is a good measure of core body temperature. But they never had an instrument with which to measure it. Now Franklin Diagnostics of Morristown, New Jersey, has developed a disposable urinary thermometer that fills that need. In a study at Hunterdon Medical Center in Flemington, New Jersey, the urinary thermometer proved more accurate than electronic instruments and as precise as mercury-in-glass thermometers.

Why a urinary thermometer? According to Joel R. L. Ehrenkrantz, M.D., who performed the study, oral temperature varies by as much as 1.6 degrees, depending on where the thermometer is placed in the mouth, and is affected by eating, drinking, smoking and talking. Rectal temperature is the highest temperature in the body, he says, and is less sensitive to fluctuations in core temperature. Add to that the embarrassment factor and the fact that glass thermometers contain toxic amounts of mercury, and you can see why Dr. Ehrenkrantz thinks the urinary thermometer should become the "method of choice" (*New Jersey Medicine*).

Patients and nurses may also prefer urinary thermometers because they save time. Dr. Ehrenkrantz estimates that a woman checking her basal body temperature each day to detect ovulation would save two hours per month.

The urinary thermometer consists of a collecting cup with a color-change sensing device that records the highest temperature during 45 seconds of immersion.

PART V: MEDICAL ADVANCES FOR A MORE BEAUTIFUL YOU

CHAPTER 23
Cosmetic Surgery: An Update

A look at new developments in the American way to save face.

"I see it as a logical extension of the health and fitness movement," Los Angeles facial surgeon Robert Kotler, M.D., says. "People have gotten their bodies in shape, now they want their faces in shape. They want to be the very best they can be."

Attitudes regarding cosmetic surgery have indeed done an about-face. Ten years ago it was only the very rich and the very vain who were having their facial structures remodeled. "Now it's anyone who wants his face to project the same vibrance as his body or his attitude," explains Dr. Kotler, coauthor of the *Consumer's Guidebook to Cosmetic Facial Surgery* (available free of charge from the American Nasal and Facial Surgery Institute, P.O. Box 97134, Los Angeles, CA 90067).

And what percentage of these alterations is being done to men? About 30 percent, reports the American Academy of Facial Plastic and Reconstructive Surgery, a 50 percent increase in the number of male clients over the past 15 years.

"Men simply are getting less reluctant to admit that it's important to them to look good," Dr. Kotler says. "What motivates a man to have cosmetic surgery nowadays isn't radically different from what motivates him to work out or buy a custom-tailored suit."

What's Available?

Facial surgery has come a long way since the days it felt pride in being able to tighten a set of drooping jowls. Here's a brief summary of what's currently possible in the hands of a competent practitioner.

The face-lift. This is the operation that gave cosmetic surgery its start, and it does precisely what it says. It lifts the skin from the face after incisions have been made just inside the hairline from the temples down to below the ears. The skin is then pulled tight and smoothed out; the excess is trimmed. Tiny stitches close the incisions, and what you're left with is a tighter fit between face and skin—especially in the area of the cheeks and neck. (The average cost is from $4,000 to $8,500, and the life expectancy of a face-lift is 10 to 12 years.)

The eye-lift. Probably the most common anti-aging operation of them all, the eye-lift focuses on excess above and below the eyes. As with the face-lift, tiny incisions are made, the skin is drawn tight (fat deposits may even be removed) and the result is a pair of eyes that are less puffy and more energetic looking. (The cost is from $1,500 to $3,500 for a job that should last 10 to 15 years.)

Dermabrasions and chemical peel. These techniques are best for wrinkles that are especially fine (such as those around the eyes and mouth), and they can be effective against acne scars as well. With dermabrasion, skin is literally sanded smooth with a high-speed wheel. With a chemical peel, a caustic compound is used that, in effect, subjects the skin to a controlled second-degree burn. With both techniques, new skin comes along to replace the old, and a smoother, more youthful appearance is the result.

Collagen injections. This technique works by smoothing wrinkles from the inside out. Collagen—a milky substance purified from cowhides—is injected beneath the skin, causing wrinkles to get pushed smooth in the style of an inflated balloon. Collagen injections work best for smile lines and wrinkled brows, but a drawback is that their effects are somewhat short-lived—only about a year or so.

Reconstructive surgery. Reconstructive surgery is facial surgery going more than skin deep. Through the reshaping of bone itself, features such as the nose, cheeks and chin can be substantially altered.

Keeping Reality in Focus

Dr. Kotler has problems with patients whose motivations stray from what's possible. "Cosmetic surgery, for a man or woman, is not in itself going to make major changes in a person's life—and it's the responsibility of a good cosmetic surgeon to let prospective clients know this. Yes, a person's attitude may become more positive as a result of his or her surgery, but that's no guarantee the person is going to get the job promotion or have a better social life," he says.

Dr. Kotler also has problems with patients wanting surgery to erase the effects of an errant lifestyle. "If a major drinker comes to me, I'll ask him to make major changes in his habit before I'll even consider surgery—not just because he may not be in good enough health to respond well, but because the surgery then becomes a guiding force, something the patient must earn. Handled in this way, facial surgery can actually help turn some people around. You give them a healthier look, but not without impressing on them that it's their responsibility to maintain it."

The Fit Recover Faster

Yet another reason to have your act together before considering facial surgery is recovery.

"It comes noticeably faster for people who are regular exercisers, eat well and don't smoke," Dr. Kotler says. "The healthier the person, the faster he heals."

And how fast is fast?

"Someone in good shape could expect total recovery—even if he or she has had multiple procedures—in two to three weeks," Dr. Kotler says. "Less extensive operations heal faster, usually in seven to ten days. Many people use vacation time."

Pushing the fitness point one step further, Dr. Kotler tells the story of one patient—a marathon runner—who saw her times drop dramatically after having her once-broken nose repaired.

"She was finally getting her RDA of oxygen," Dr. Kotler says.

CHAPTER 24

The Modern War on Baldness

Why live bald if you don't want to? Despite a long history of hucksterism, today's new rugs, plugs and drugs offer a wide range of alternatives.

In early 1983, Elaine Orenburg, Ph.D., a Stanford University cell biologist, took the usual steps to find subjects for what seemed like a routine experiment. She asked the Stanford Public Information Service to place a request for volunteers in the student newspaper. Dr. Orenburg planned to test minoxidil, an experimental drug reputed to grow hair on balding heads. The PR people, sensing a news angle, asked her permission to notify some off-campus media. Dr. Orenberg said, "Sure," and didn't give the matter a second thought—until the phones began ringing.

"Within one hour, every phone line into dermatology was jammed," she recalls. "We received more than 1,000 calls within two weeks and turned away hundreds of men who besieged the office when they couldn't get through by phone."

The same thing happened to Ronald Savin, M.D., a dermatologist at Yale—only much worse. Dr. Savin was also about to test the drug that had grown "significant" hair on one-third of balding men in pilot studies. His request for volunteers was picked up by the wire services.

"My phone went absolutely crazy," he says. "My regular patients couldn't get through for a month. Men called from all over the country dying to volunteer. It was incredible."

Youth and Virility

Ever since Samson lost his strength when he lost his hair, balding has implied a great deal more to men than simply the need to use sunscreen on top of their heads at the beach. "Balding is the hammerlock that mortality holds on men's conceits," Jeff Shear wrote in the "About Men" column of the *New York Times Magazine*. "It is the final takedown in the fight to stay youthful." Shear's hair loss made him feel "self-conscious, diminished, vulnerable and alarmed." Dr. Savin, who calls himself "moderately bald" despite minoxidil and hair transplants, says that hair is "terribly important to men's self-esteem. A full head of hair has always implied youth, confidence and vitality."

For men in their thirties and forties today, it often implies even more. This is the generation brought up on President Kennedy's bushy locks, Edd "Kookie" Byrnes lending his comb, the "mop-top" Beatles, and even a hit musical and movie entitled—what else?—*Hair:* "Give me a head with hair, long beautiful hair. . . . There ain't no words for the beauty, the splendor, the wonder of my hair."

In *The Doctor's Book on Hair Loss,* T. Gerald Aldhizer, M.D., recounts his sadness at joining what he ruefully calls The Club. "My father warned me about it. It's an outfit nobody wants to belong to, with dues nobody wants to pay—expensive dues: depression, embarrassment and loss of self-confidence. My mirror became my enemy."

This sentiment has been echoed throughout recorded history. As early as 4,000 B.C., the Egyptians were rubbing balding scalps with a concoction of dates, ground animal parts and oil. Ever since then, "baldness cures" have ranked right up there with aphrodisiacs and weight-loss elixirs as staples of medical hucksterism. In January 1985, the U.S. Food and Drug Administration (FDA) banned all over-the-counter hair-growth lotions as "useless."

Yet the hair replacement industry is healthier than ever. Open any men's magazine or newspaper sports or business section and you're likely to find advertisements for prescription hair-growth lotions, cosmetic surgery and several different types of hairpieces. Those in the field say that millions of men are desperate to escape being called Skinhead, Chrome Dome, Baldy, and Billiard Ball. No one knows how large the hair restoration market is, but those who follow it are quick to say, "billions."

Some women say that bald is sexy, and advice columnists reassure men that what's inside the head is more important than what's on top of it. But the macho images of Yul Brynner and Telly Savalas are cold comfort to the millions of men who start each day carefully plastering their remaining hair over growing bald spots.

Age, Heredity, and Hormones

There are two kinds of hair, vellus and terminal. The former is often called peach fuzz. The latter is what two-thirds of men (and 10 percent of women) regret losing.

Hair grows in three stages. During the anagen phase, which lasts for three to five years, hair grows about ½ inch per month. About 85 percent of the hair is in the anagen phase. Then comes the ten-day catagen phase, when the blood supply to the hair root decreases and the hair stops growing. Finally, during the four- to six-month telogen

(continued on page 168)

One in Ten: Women and Hair Loss

If you think *men* get upset about losing their hair, try raising the subject with a balding *woman.*

"A few days after I started my freshman year at college," 35-year-old Ashley Siegel recalls, "I awoke with a burning sensation on my scalp. On my pillow lay huge clumps of hair. In the shower, more hair fell out. I thought I was hallucinating. I'll never forget the look on the dermatologist's face when he told me I was going to lose all my hair. He said I had alopecia areata, and that there was no cure. He advised me to buy a wig and get on with my life as best I could.

"My first thought was that no one could know about this. I put every ounce of my strength into keeping my horrible secret. I couldn't bear to see myself without my wig. I slept with it on. I took showers at 2:00 A.M. so no one could see me. I lived in terror of a strong wind."

Alopecia areata, an autoimmune disease in which the body mistakes its own hair-root cells for foreign invaders and destroys them, afflicts 250,000 Americans, many of them women. Although there is no cure, vitamin and mineral supplements, minoxidil and other drugs often spur regrowth.

"With aggressive treatment, about 60 percent of our areata patients get regrowth," says Wilma F. Bergfeld, M.D., a Cleveland Clinic Foundation dermatologist. "But it's a chemically recurring problem. You've got to follow it closely."

Alopecia areata is just one reason that 10 percent of women experience noticeable hair loss. Like many men, some women are genetically predisposed to pattern baldness along the hairline and at the crown, but female pattern hair loss is usually much less extensive. The hormonal mechanism is similar—both sexes produce androgens—but in women the key hormone is dihydroepiandosterone sulfate (DHEAS), according to dermatologist Joel Kassimer, M.D., of New York University Medical Center.

Other causes of hair loss in women include the drugs and illnesses mentioned in the chapter text; "traction alopecia," from pulling ponytails too tight; chemical damage from overuse of hair dyes; and pregnancy, childbirth, menopause and birth control pills, because of the hormonal changes they cause.

"Hair loss is surprisingly common among women," Dr. Bergfeld says. "I'm 48 and have lost some as a result of menopause. But no one would know because of the way I wear my hair. I'm all for cosmetic restyling and anything else that preserves women's self-esteem."

"Most women experience some hair loss as they grow older," says Dr. Kassimer. "About 10 percent suffer significant loss, but you have to lose about 50 percent in any area for it to become obvious. Hairdressing can help quite a bit. So can hairpieces, transplants and minoxidil."

The tragedy is that female hair loss is virtually unmentionable. Few women realize it's possible, and those who suffer significant hair loss rarely understand their alternatives or receive adequate support. "It was my deep, dark secret," recalls a 33-year-old New York City publicist who was helped by Pilo-Genic Research Associates, a hair-loss clinic in New York. "I have pretty nice hair again—not as full as before, but noticeably improved. I got my problem under control seven years ago, but for years I never discussed my secret with my husband. Finally I told him last year. I could hardly get the words out. He was understanding, but the whole subject still makes me very uncomfortable."

phase, the hair falls out. About 12 percent of hair is in the telogen phase. Each scalp hair is genetically programmed to grow—and stop growing—individually.

Hair fallout is perfectly normal. The typical adult loses about 75 hairs a day. These usually grow back unless the person's age, heredity and hormones conspire to shut down the hair follicles, in which case terminal hair gives way to vellus hair, then nothing.

Hair "thinning" is often used synonymously with hair loss, but the two are different. Even if hair does not fall out, each strand becomes physically thinner with age. Both men's and women's hair loses about 5 percent of its thickness from age 20 to 50 and another 15 percent from age 50 to 80.

The most common form of hair loss is male pattern baldness (MPB), or androgenic alopecia. The hairline recedes. A bald spot appears on the back of the head (the crown). Then the two hairless areas meet and expand until the man is left with just a "horseshoe fringe" of vellus hair.

"Years ago, we believed that MPB was a sex-linked genetic trait," says Joel Kassimir, M.D., a clinical instructor of dermatology at New York University Medical Center. "If a man's maternal grandfather was bald, the theory was that he would be, too. But now we know that balding is not that simple. It can be inherited from both parents and does not pass uniformly to children. In many families, one son goes bald and another does not. There are probably several genes for hair loss that get turned on by several other factors."

If a man has a genetic predisposition to MPB, actual hair loss will depend on his age and male sex hormones (androgens). "The age factor comes down to the '10 Percent Rule,' " Dr. Kassimir says. "Ten percent of men show obvious hair loss in their teens, 20 percent in their twenties and so on. Hair loss can start at any age, but the earlier it begins, the more severe it is likely to be. Men who become substantially bald usually show significant loss by age 35."

In MPB, the hormone that influences hair loss, dihydrotestosterone (DHT), is created when testosterone circulating in the blood encounters the enzyme 5-alpha-reductase.

Some hair follicles have genetically programmed receptor sites for DHT receptors and continue to produce terminal hair even if they are moved to bald areas—hence hair transplantation.

Balding has been linked to testosterone ever since 400 B.C., when Hippocrates observed that eunuchs, who lack testosterone-producing testicles, never go bald. Hair loss was once thought to relate to "excess" testosterone. Since testosterone is popularly associated with masculinity and male sexuality, there was a time when bald men were considered "more sexual," since their baldness indicated that they had excess testosterone. This idea was wrong on two counts. First, the body needs only a tiny amount of testosterone to ensure a normal male (or female) sex drive. Any extra testosterone has no effect on sexuality. And second, hair loss has nothing to do with testosterone per se, but rather with its derivative, DHT, and with the person's genetic heritage.

In addition to age, heredity and DHT, many other factors can also cause balding. Drugs are a big factor in hair loss. Antidepressants, amphetamines, hormones, anticoagulants and drugs prescribed for cancer, heart disease and high blood pressure frequently cause temporary hair loss. Hair regenerates after use of the offending drug is terminated.

Significant hair loss may also result from the stress of physical or emotional trauma, according to Wilma F. Bergfeld, M.D., a dermatologist at the Cleveland Clinic Foundation. Within four to six weeks of the triggering event—high fever, childbirth, general anesthesia or emotional turmoil, among others—25 to 50 percent of hair may fall out.

Several illnesses also cause hair loss, particularly alopecia areata, a poorly understood autoimmune disease that afflicts about 250,000 people in the United States. Ringworm of the scalp (tinea capitis, a fungal infection) also causes significant hair shedding. Hair loss may also result from anorexia nervosa. Hair is composed of protein. When a person starves, the body shuts down such biologically marginal activities as hair production and channels all available protein to more vital functions.

Rugs

"Mention hair replacement, and people immediately think of the worthless potions the FDA recently banned," says Mary-Ellen Siegel, author of *Reversing Hair Loss*. "The fact is, if you have the money, there are reasonably good alternatives for just about everyone. Nothing is perfect, but you don't have to live bald if you don't want to."

The classic approach is the hairpiece. Toupees, or "rugs," were once embarrassingly obvious, but no longer. Good hairpieces, which cost from $500 to $1,200, are lightweight (no more than a few ounces), don't feel hot, adhere well and look natural (which means that extra care is taken with the hairline). The heavy cotton and rubber foundations of yesteryear have given way to light, sheer nylon mesh. The hair itself may be either synthetic or natural (usually from Italian women) or a combination of both. Natural hair looks and dyes better, but it dries more slowly, tangles more easily and doesn't hold up as well as the synthetics. Several adhesives are available, but the type most widely recommended is hypoallergenic, double-facing tape. Tape provides generally reliable adhesion but may fail during strenuous exercise, or under water, or if pulled. Most hairpieces must be professionally cleaned annually and replaced every few years.

A different kind of hairpiece, known as a hair extension, has been popularized by Hair Club for Men (HCM), which has eight centers around the country. Unlike standard hairpieces, HCM's creations can go anywhere, a point emphasized relentlessly in the company's brochures, which depict satisfied customers swimming, running, playing tennis, showering and allowing women to run their fingers through their new hair. The key is HCM's attachment system, tiny nylon threads that extend from the hairpiece and are tied to the man's (or woman's) remaining hair. Of course, HCM's heavy-duty hairpieces come at a heavy-duty price, $1,800 to $3,200, plus $60 per visit for "snug-ups" every two months, during which the anchor lines are tightened. "HCM is a good choice for the younger, more active man who doesn't want to worry about the limitations of standard hairpieces," Siegel says. "He can play racquetball, then jump in the shower, then towel- or blow-dry and drive his convertible to pick up his date with no problem."

Plugs

Surgical hair replacement dates from 1950, when Norman Orentreich, M.D., a clinical professor of dermatology at New York University Medical Center and one of the nation's foremost hair researchers, performed the first successful hair transplant. Since then, more than two million North American men and women have had hair transplants. A local anesthetic numbs the scalp, then the surgeon uses a small instrument (an Orentreich punch) to remove plugs of hair-bearing scalp and stamp them into bald scalp. The number of transplantable plugs depends on the amount of remaining hair. If more than half the live follicles in any area are transplanted, the donor area looks denuded. Transplanted hair typically falls out shortly after being moved, but new terminal hair almost always grows back. Transplants typically cost about $20 to $25 per plug. Fifty to 200 plugs are typically transplanted at a cost of $1,000 to $5,000. (Health insurance rarely covers the procedure.)

"Before you agree to hair transplants," Dr. Kassimir recommends, "be sure to see 'before' and 'after' pictures of the surgeon's patients. The hair should look natural with no 'corn row effect'—discernible lines of wefts. Pay particular attention to the hairline. The only way to get a truly natural-looking hairline is to transplant single hairs, but many dermatologists don't do this. About half my transplant practice is devoted to correcting other surgeons' bad work."

Another surgical approach, scalp reduction, is similar to a face-lift. Skin, including the scalp, is elastic, but as it ages, it tends to sag, most noticeably into facial wrinkles and double chins, which face-lifting largely eliminates by pulling sagging skin tighter. Scalp reduction uses the same principle. The surgeon removes an oval-shaped section of scalp from the top of the head, then pulls the hair-bearing scalp below it upward to cover more of the head. Scalp reduction leaves a scar along the top of the head, which remains bald, so the procedure is usually followed by hair transplants or a hairpiece. But for men who have only horseshoe rings left, scalp reduction provides better coverage with less surgery than hair transplantation by itself. Scalp reduction costs about $2,000.

Scalp expansion is the latest wrinkle, as it were, in skin stretching. Small balloons are surgically inserted into the scalp above the ears. Over several weeks, the balloons are filled with saline solution. As the balloons expand, so does the scalp that covers them. During the expansion phase, the head looks deformed, so the person undergoing the procedure usually wants to keep his head covered. Once the scalp has been expanded, it is pulled up to cover the bald area. Since scalp expansion occurs more gradually than scalp reduction, it can be used to cover large bald areas and tends to cover more evenly. It costs $3,000 to $4,500.

Hair-Regrowth Lotions

Despite the recent FDA ban on over-the-counter hair-growth products, two prescription hair restorers, biotin and minoxidil, are quite popular—and controversial. Biotin is a B vitamin. When taken orally, it has no effect on human hair, but during the 1960s, Edward Settel, M.D., a New York gerontologist who had been experimenting with hair restorers, became intrigued by reports that biotin helped thicken fur-bearing animals' coats. He theorized that biotin could prevent hair follicles from binding DHT and dying if it could penetrate to the root of the hair. After experimenting with several lotion formulas that did not reach all the way to the hair root, Dr. Settel patented a deep-penetrating "mini-emulsion" which, he claimed, bathed the hair root in enough biotin to displace bound DHT and regrow some balding men's hair. In 1971, he founded Pilo-Genic Research Associates in New York,

which today boasts 67 physician-supervised clinics around the country. Anita Young, Dr. Settel's wife, who became company president after her husband's death in 1984, says Pilo-Genic grossed $8 million in 1985.

Does biotin work? That is a matter of passionately divided opinion. Young makes no claim that it works for everyone. She says the best candidates are men under 40 who are losing their hair but are not yet bald. The longer the man has been bald, the less effective biotin becomes. Overall, she says, "more than half of those who still have functioning follicles get significant results without side effects." But most dermatologists scoff at this claim. Dr. Stavin calls Pilo-Genic "snake oil." Dr. Kassimir says, "There are no hard data to show that it works. Many of my patients have tried it unsuccessfully."

The FDA investigated Pilo-Genic in 1975, 1976 and 1977, based on a Detroit user's complaint of false advertising. The FDA found no cause for action. This finding does not constitute an endorsement of Pilo-Genic; it simply means that the agency had no objections to its advertising claims.

In 1984, Pilo-Genic sponsored a year-long double-blind test. Young says, "Seventy-seven percent of the men treated with our product experienced significant hair regrowth." But critics counter that the results of such tests are open to manipulation. They want Pilo-Genic's formula tested like minoxidil at major medical centers. A spokesman for Hill Top Research, the laboratory near Cincinnati that conducted the biotin test, declined comment on the results. Young says that unlike Upjohn, the company that produces minoxidil, Pilo-Genic is too small to underwrite extensive testing at major medical centers.

To date, the only clinical test of Pilo-Genic was a two-year, double-blind pilot study by Dr. Bergfeld at the Cleveland Clinic. "Of the 20 men, 3 grew vellus hair," she says. "None grew terminal hair. Still, I was impressed. I have patients who were not in my study who say that Pilo-Genic has helped them grow hair."

"It's worked great for me," says Reverend John Gregory Tweed, a 46-year-old New York psychotherapist. "I had only a fringe left, and they told me that biotin might not work. But I was willing to spend the $150 for the exam and a few months of lotion. First, I got some peach fuzz. Then I started to grow real hair. Over time, I regained quite a bit. I still have a receded hairline and a bald spot on my crown, but I have enough on top to part my hair. Pilo-Genic has taken ten years off my looks and all for just $1.25 a day."

Pilo-Genic's clientele, once completely male, is now 35 percent female. The initial exam costs $75. The lotion and shampoo cost $40 a month. Even critics say biotin is harmless. Young says that those who respond generally achieve maximum results within two years at a cost of about $1,400.

Despite testimonials, Pilo-Genic's lack of clinical research and the company's franchise-clinic organization have relegated biotin to the medical fringe and kept dermatologists—and millions of balding men and women—searching for The Ultimate Cure. Some say that minoxidil just might be it.

Breakthrough?

Minoxidil is the active ingredient in Upjohn's Loniten, a blood-vessel-expanding antihypertensive drug approved by the FDA in 1979. Years earlier, physicians testing it had noticed that it also stimulated the growth of body hair. They alerted some research dermatologists, who approached the drug company about investigating a minoxidil lotion for hair restoration. Upjohn quietly tested several formulations, then in 1983 launched the study of 2,300 balding volunteers at 28 medical centers that jammed so many phone lines.

Yale's Dr. Savin calls minoxidil "a real breakthrough. It's the first thing that isn't snake oil." His results generally agree with those of Dr. Kassimir in New York and Dr. Bergfeld in Cleveland: "About 10 percent of men get bushy growth; 30 percent grow some terminal hair; 30 percent get peach fuzz and the rest grow nothing. The best regrowth occurs on the crown. Minoxidil does not work as well along the hairline."

Both Dr. Savin and Dr. Kassimir use minoxidil themselves. "The bald spot I used to have on my crown is now covered with two-inch hairs," Dr. Kassimir says. "I have hair transplants, and minoxidil acts like fertilizer," Dr. Savin says.

At the 2 percent concentration in the experimental solutions, minoxidil causes "virtually no side effects," researchers agree. (Do not use higher concentrations, however. Side effects may occur.) A few users get scalp rashes, which appear to be caused by the other ingredients in the lotion.

But there's a big problem with minoxidil even for the lucky few who grow lots of hair. Once the user stops applying the lotion, any new hair falls out within a few months.

"I prescribe minoxidil," hair-transplant pioneer Dr. Orentreich says. "It opens up exciting new avenues for research. But I'm not a fan of it. It's not a 'breakthrough.' At best, it's a 'mini-breakthrough.' My results have not been as good as some other researchers'. Among my subjects, only 1 in 500 has grown bushy hair. One percent have grown some terminal hair, and 10 percent have gotten peach fuzz, but most wound up with little beyond disappointment. And even the few who get good growth lose their new hair when they stop using it."

But as far as the balding public is concerned, Dr. Orentreich is, well, splitting hairs. Upjohn declines to release sales figures, but securities analysts estimate that since minoxidil testing began, Loniten sales have quadrupled from an estimated $10 million to more than $40 million, with as much as 95 percent of the increase finding its way onto balding heads. "Many people have persuaded their physicians to prescribe Loniten; then they take it to a pharmacy and have it made into an ointment," Dr. Savin says. Neither Upjohn nor the FDA approves of "extemporaneous use of experimental drugs," but clearly, many physicians have been unable to say no.

Beyond Minoxidil

Other drug companies are hot on Upjohn's trail. Lederle Laboratories is currently conducting clinical trials of a possible hair-raiser called Viprostol at nine medical centers around the country. Like minoxidil, Viprostol is a vasodilator; it increases blood flow to the skin. One theory of balding holds that the DHT that binds to hair follicles destined to die does not kill them outright, but rather shuts off blood circulation. By restoring lost blood flow, Lederle researchers hope to restore hair as well.

Another purported hair restorer, Nutriol, is produced by an Italian drug company, Crinos International, and marketed in the United States by a network of independent distributors. Nutriol, known in Europe as Foltene, is licensed in France, Italy, Greece and a few other countries as a hair restorer, based on nine clinical studies performed by scientists in France and Italy, which Crinos promotional materials say showed "significant hair restoration." It has never been tested in the United States.

Does Nutriol work? Dr. Bergfeld says its formula "has never been shown to grow hair." However, William Holloway, M.D., a 62-year-old psychiatrist in Hemet, California, says it has helped him grow "significant hair" on his crown. Dr. Holloway says he was so impressed that his wife has become a Nutriol distributor. He says the product works for about 70 percent of those who use it, but that, as with minoxidil, new hair falls out once the product's use is discontinued.

Nutriol is officially a cosmetic hair conditioner and, as a cosmetic, the FDA allows it into the United States. It cannot be advertised as a hair restorer, but it's impossible for the FDA to prevent Nutriol distributors from telling their customers that it grows hair. Dr. Holloway, whose wife distributes the product, says distributors make no hair-restoration claims, but it's difficult to believe that so many men would shell out hundreds of dollars for a mere hair conditioner.

Nutriol contains all 22 amino acids, biotin and various other vitamins and a dizzying array of other chemicals, including mucopolysaccharides, key ingredients that Crinos says nourish hair follicles. In the words of Dr. Bergfeld, "They've put everything in there but the kitchen sink." Users apply one vial of Nutriol to the scalp every other day for 24 applications, then use one or two vials a week for six months. Total cost: $500 to $800.

Bald Is Beautiful

Although millions of men spend billions a year to replace their lost locks, John T. Capps III spends his money doing the opposite—promoting baldness. The 46-year-old North Carolina printer is the founder and president of the 15,000-member organization Bald-Headed Men of America (BHMA). Capps says, "I'm proud of every hair I don't have. If you haven't got it, flaunt it." Capps began losing his hair in high school and recalls being teased mercilessly by his schoolmates. "Now they're all bald and miserable, while I'm happy as can be." Capps's secret? "Positive attitude. I accept myself as I am. I like how I look. And I enjoy a good laugh—even at my own expense." Capps spends his time touring the talk shows in his station wagon (his license plate reads "BALD 1"), spreading the gospel of Happy Hairlessness. "BHMA has nothing against men who use minoxidil or get hairpieces or transplants, but we're not into drugs, rugs or plugs. We like to meet our problems head on. We say, 'Skin is in.' The good Lord created only a few perfect heads. The rest he covered with hair."

CHAPTER 25

Seeing Better, Looking Younger: A Breakthrough in Eye Care

The latest advances in bifocal contact lenses may make it possible for many to shed their age-revealing eyeglasses.

There's nothing quite like bifocal eyeglasses to signal that you're part of the "old guard"—and it's not always a flattering shift in image. Who really wants to acknowledge the aging process in such a visible manner?

That's particularly true if you've been able to wear contact lenses up to now, because bifocal contacts just haven't worked well for most patients. A *New York Times* report estimates that, because bifocal contacts are troublesome to fit and make, "as many as four of every five people who try to wear them go back to spectacles."

Fortunately, two companies have developed what they believe are soft bifocal contacts that can work—not only for comfortable wear but for better vision. More than 70 percent of the patients who tried the two new lenses in clinical tests were able to wear them. That's good news for bifocal wearers, who, with trifocal wearers, make up half of all Americans needing eyeglasses or contacts.

How the New Bifocal Contacts Work

Up to now, bifocal contacts have had "translating" lenses that move around on your eye with the help of your lower eyelid. The shifts in movement are needed to bring the right optical field in place so you can see, whether for distance vision or reading.

If you have astigmatism, hard translating lenses are actually the best fitting, but people with normally shaped eyes find soft lenses better. The new contacts, both soft, use simultaneous lenses that don't need to move around. Instead, the reading and distance optics are put before the retina at the same time. Your brain can select which focus you need and ignore the others—a process identical to what happens in normal vision.

Each of the new lenses—which may not be available yet for purchase—uses further refinements to aid your vision. The ALGES lens, made by University Optical Products, puts the optics in a bull's-eye pattern on the lens. The reading portion of the lens is in the center and the distance lens is on the outer circumference. The arrangement is closest to the way your eye works naturally.

The Hydrocurve II, produced by Barnes-Hind, is a multifocal lens that corrects your vision at intermediate points as well as near and distant points. The back surface of the lens is curved to allow just such "blended" vision. Both the Hydrocurve II and the ALGES lens make use of laser technology to produce more exact lens cuttings—in fact, because the ALGES lens's cutting directions are computer stored, any of 984 bifocal prescriptions can be recreated on demand, according to its maker, University Optical.

Adjusting to Bifocals: Patience and Perspective

It's important to remember that even bifocal contacts won't be perfect once they're on the market—just as their eyeglass counterparts aren't. "There are 100 million pairs of bifocal spectacles prescribed each year, and the people who wear them sometimes trip down steps or can't read the top of a newspaper," noted one contact-lens expert in an interview with the *New York Times*. "But the bottom line is that they work. Bifocal contact lenses also have problems, but just as with spectacles, it's sometimes a compromise."

Despite your concerns over how bifocals will make you look, your vision needs are more important. Until the new lens configurations are available, you may have to wear the more obvious spectacles and adjust your habits and viewpoint accordingly. If that's the case, you can make the adjustment easier on yourself in a few simple ways.

First, take the time to discuss your needs carefully with your optometrist, whether you're about to get spectacles or hard contact lenses. Ask him or her to describe in detail the problems or discomfort that your particular vision needs may cause as you adjust physically to your prescription. And keep track of those problems. It's common for bifocal contact-lens wearers to see "ghost images" for the first week or two. You'll appear much more natural with glasses or contacts if you don't need to continually adjust them at work.

Second, choose your frames with care—particularly if you've never had to wear glasses before and if the change in image is already unnerving you. Attractive frames can go a long way to dispel your worries about looking older and can even add to your appearance.

Finally, realize that half of the image battle lies in your viewpoint. If you can stride into work wearing bifocal spectacles with an air of confidence, chances are that few people will notice them—and those who do will tailor their comments to your apparent comfort or discomfort with them.

CHAPTER 26
Science against Scars

With a little help from recent research, you may be able to prevent or erase an ugly scar.

Scarred for life—a terrifying thought. Scars are the mainstay of horror and gangster films; the volatile fuel of nightmares. Who can forget the Frankenstein monster's ghoulish railroad-track scars or the disfigurement of the gangster Scarface?

To most people, scars are unrelenting reminders of accidents, injuries or surgical trauma. They can be psychologically debilitating. Disfigurement can force a person to be repeatedly confronted with embarrassing wide-eyed stares, insensitive questions and cruel remarks. Such has been the experience of A. J., a UCLA graduate student who was severely burned by an accident with a home barbecue at age nine. He suffered tremendous teasing throughout childhood. Even as an adult, A. J. suffers the stares and comments of insensitive people. "I saw 'A. J. the Burned' written on one of the tables in a classroom at UCLA," he confides softly. "It made me feel terrible. It means someone sees me only as my scars."

Surgical patients as well as accident victims experience great distress over scarring. "People are more concerned with scarring than any other aspect of surgery," says Eugene Weinstein, M.D., a general surgeon in North Hollywood, California. "Before surgery, all they ask is 'What kind of scar am I going to have? How long will it be?' "

A study at the University of Pennsylvania Cancer Center showed that people who accurately anticipated their scar size prior to surgery were significantly less distressed by their scar's appearance than those whose scars were larger than they'd expected. Without presurgical counseling to help them adjust, some people feel overwhelmed when they see their scars.

John, a computer programmer in Gaithersburg, Maryland, never had time to anticipate his scars. He was rushed into emergency surgery after a serious football knee injury. "I started to think about my scar just before I got my cast off. I figured I'd have a little scar, a thin white line," explains John. "When I saw it, I was shocked at how big it was; really thick, wide and long. You could still see the holes from the stitches."

Scar Formation

A scar, medically known as a cicatrix, is a defect that remains in the skin after a wound heals. A healing wound goes through three stages: inflammation, healing and scar formation. During the inflammatory phase, blood fluid (plasma), platelets, and fibrin, a filamentlike protein, accumulate in the wound. The platelets and fibrin form a blood clot and weakly hold the wound edges together for four to six days.

After the sixth day, the healing phase begins. New connective tissue forms, adding strength and flexibility to the healing wound.

During scar formation, connective collagen fibers tightly link together to increase strength as the wound contracts and closes. This process may take 3 to 12 months. The result is a scar, a whitish, glistening area that settles either slightly above or below the skin surface.

Scar types and appearance vary. In some wounds, excess collagen becomes trapped within the wound and produces a wide, thick (hypertrophic) scar. Severe burns tend to form hypertrophic scars due to the prolonged inflammatory phase and the subsequent increase in collagen formation. However, pressure from an elastic bandage applied over a healing burn may prevent or retard this collagen buildup and reduce scar size.

An excessive accumulation of collagen outside the wound results in a thicker scar called a keloid. The tissue healing response becomes exaggerated, and scar tissue overwhelms the wound. The result is an unsightly, raised, red or purple scar that contains blood vessels. A keloid may feel sensitive and continue to grow for a prolonged period. John's surgical knee scar developed into a keloid. "It is still dark purple. Even after 12 years, only the ends of the scar have begun to fade," he says. "It's itchy and very sensitive." The tendency to develop keloid scars appears to be inherited. Blacks, Asians and people with olive or freckled skin are most susceptible.

Scarring Complications

A variety of factors can disrupt the normal healing process and produce abnormal, irregular scarring. A heavier scar may result from excessive movement or tension due to the wound's location. The outside of the upper arm, once the preferred site for immunizations, typically produces large scars due to frequent stretching of the skin. Some authorities now suggest immunizations be given on the upper inner arm to produce less scarring. The chest and upper back are also prone to large scars due to skin tension.

But regardless of the wound location, Dr. Weinstein says, "Scarring is an individual matter. There is no way to predict how you'll heal. How you scar in one area has no relation to how you heal in another."

Certain first aid measures may disrupt normal healing processes. Steroid creams and alcohol solutions may delay healing. Anti-inflammatory drugs suppress the wound repair process. And prolonged antibiotic use can increase the risk of skin infection and delay healing by encouraging the development of resistant bacteria strains. Similarly, exposing fresh wounds to the air dehydrates tissues and interferes with rebuilding. To prevent air exposure, severe burns should be covered with temporary natural or manmade "skins" while awaiting skin-grafting procedures.

Contrary to popular belief, topical vitamin E has adverse effects on healing. According to Robert L. Ruberg, M.D., associate professor of surgery at Ohio State University, vitamin E interferes with collagen synthesis much like steroids do. Vitamin E is being used, however, to retard the excessive growth of keloids or hypertrophic scars.

Obesity also poses problems for proper tissue repair. Fatty tissue has a limited blood supply. Wounds in fatty areas may become infected more easily. Fat is also more difficult to suture. The skin around the injured area can become stressed, which delays healing and aggravates scar formation.

Finally, smokers have a reduced ability to heal wounds properly because of reduced oxygen circulating in the blood. This lack of oxygen can seriously hinder tissue regeneration.

Scar Self-Care

Several factors can influence scarring. Good nutrition and proper care of injuries can accelerate healing and minimize scarring.

Vitamins. Substantial biochemical research suggests that nutrition plays a vital role in the healing process. Vitamins A, B, C and K all aid in cell growth, assist enzyme formation and foster blood clotting, all of which contribute to infection resistance and healing. Vitamin A also counteracts the inhibitory effect of steroid therapy on the healing process. Vitamin C in particular plays an important role in healing. A deficiency of vitamin C can alter the healing process and disrupt collagen synthesis. A person deficient in vitamin C not only may be unable to heal new wounds properly but may also find that old wounds reopen.

Minerals. The minerals zinc, copper and iron assist in connective tissue formation, strengthening wound repair.

In addition, the amino acid methionine may accelerate the development of connective tissue (fibroplasia) and reduce the length of the inflammatory phase. It's debatable whether amino acid supplementation accelerates healing. But a diet lacking in protein impairs healing. Make sure your diet has enough.

First aid. When managing minor injuries at home, several things can be done to reduce tissue trauma and decrease scar severity. To clean a fresh wound, use an antibacterial skin cleanser such as povidone-iodine solution or ordinary white soap (without additives or fragrances), and rinse well with clean water. If a wound is deep or contaminated by dirt and debris, use a turkey baster or similar tool to force a stream of water through it for adequate flushing. If further scrubbing is necessary, use cotton rather than gauze to control irritation and cell damage.

Regardless of the injury (including burns), always dress a wound to promote healing. Covering exposed, damaged tissue speeds healing by preventing dehydration. A hydrated wound is less painful, and scar formation is minimized. Select a material such as Telfa, available in drugstores, which absorbs excess blood and fluid without dehydrating the wound and does not stick to the tissue. Dry cotton and gauze fibers can become trapped in the scab and stick to bare wounds. Telfa has a plastic film that allows absorption but keeps fiber from invading the wound.

Burns. Burns need special care. They require prompt, correct action. First-degree burns—sunburns, for example—are minor. Second-degree burns, such as serious sunburns or burns caused by contact with hot liquids, are more serious. They are persistently painful, appear red or mottled and may have a wet, weepy appearance. Third-degree burns are commonly caused by fire or electricity. They have a pale or charred appearance, with broken skin and a dry surface. Third-degree burns are not painful because the nerves in the burned tissues have been destroyed. These burns can lead to fluid loss and serious infection. Seek medical attention immediately.

Treating a burn correctly at home can reduce scarring and prevent infection. Susan Jackson, head nurse in the burn unit at Santa Clara Valley Hospital in San Jose, California, advises against using home remedies such as butter or aloe vera, which may further damage burned tissue. Most minor burns should be immersed in cold water for several minutes. She also warns against breaking blisters or peeling skin. Blisters, nature's Band-Aids, provide sterile protection and should be left intact. If a blister breaks, flush the wound with clean water and apply a fresh bandage.

Marine injuries. Like burns, marine injuries require special attention. Contrary to popular belief, the salt in ocean water does not sterilize an open wound. Instead, it may encourage infection by more than 20 known salt-loving human pathogens. To reduce the possibility of infection, carefully irrigate the wound and apply an antibacterial ointment such as Betadine.

Sweet Solutions

In addition to the self-care strategies already mentioned, honey can be a valuable antiscarring addition to your medicine cabinet. The medicinal use of honey is widely accepted in folk medicine. Honey has been used for wound healing since early Egyptian times. Russian soldiers used honey to aid healing during World War I. Now modern medicine is finally recognizing honey's healing properties. A clinical study reported in the *American Journal of Surgery* supports honey's ability to promote and accelerate wound healing. Honey is nontoxic, hypoallergenic, easily acquired and an inexpensive topical ointment for home use. Commercial unboiled honey is composed of simple sugars, water, amino acids, vitamins, minerals and enzymes, all vital to proper healing. In addition to providing an excellent source of energy and enzymes for growing tissue, it reduces the buildup of fluid in the injured tissues. It also provides a barrier to bacteria and prevents dehydration.

According to Richard A. Knutson, M.D., of the Delta Orthopedic Clinic in Greenville, Mississippi, "The history of healing with sugar is widespread. High levels of sugar significantly inhibit bacterial reproduction." Dr. Knutson has developed a sugar salve that he has successfully used on more than 3,000 patients, including 800 burn cases. "We've used it successfully on all areas of the body," he reports. In eight years he has performed only five skin grafts, a figure he attributes to his salve. "Scarring is very minimal," says Dr. Knutson. "Our results are comparable to or better looking than skin grafts."

Surgical Scars

Surgical incisions present unique circumstances for healing and scar formation. The force required to close the wound directly relates to the eventual appearance of the scar. Even the direction of the incision affects the scar's appearance. Over the years, surgical techniques have evolved into incisions that follow the body's natural creases, minimizing tension and camouflaging the scar in skin folds or hairlines.

A Caesarean section, for example, can be accomplished through a vertical, midline incision. However, an improved understanding of wound healing and tissue tension has resulted in the much less conspicuous, horizontal "bikini" incision along the pubic hairline. Plastic surgeons have their patients smile, frown and grimace in order to find lines where incisions may be hidden. In many cases, a surgeon can offer some latitude in planning the incision to provide a less conspicuous scar. These aesthetic compromises, however, may complicate some procedures due to decreased accessibility of target tissues and increased anesthesia time.

In closing a surgical incision, the main consideration is preventing infection, but the surgeon should try to restrict scar formation and create a cosmetically acceptable scar. An informal survey of 90 surgeons from various specialties at a southern California hospital showed that 80 percent felt they use stitching (suturing) techniques that provide the best results both medically and aesthetically. "I'm aware of my aesthetic responsibilities," asserts Dr. Weinstein. "I use the finest suture materials possible and take out the sutures as soon as possible."

However, talk with your surgeon about your scar before surgery. Information should include the site of the incision and any site options, the type of closure material and the scar's probable appearance. Presurgical instructions should also include photographs of patients with similar scars. Patients should receive after-care instructions tailored for their suture material and incision location.

Among the most successful surgical closure materials are absorbable sutures placed under the skin (subcuticular tissue). Another method, the Allis closure, does not use skin sutures. Several clamps are placed along the incision until it has closed. The clamps are then removed and a sticky spray is applied along with tape strips to complete the closure. When applicable, the Allis closure is superior to subcuticular stitches because most tissue reacts unfavorably to suture material. "Not only does patient comfort increase with the Allis closure," according to Dr. Weinstein, "but skin stitch infections are eliminated, and people are able to shower as soon as they want. It's especially good for kids."

Scar Wars

When proper care is not enough to prevent or decrease undesirable scarring, there are several ways to make scars look more attractive (scar revision).

Steroid injections. These can suppress the regenerative ability of a scar's cells, slowing down an overreactive (hypertrophic) scar.

Laser treatment. The carbon dioxide laser can vaporize scar tissue and reduce the possibility of regrowth.

Cryosurgery. This method, which is the application of freezing liquid nitrogen, is an alternative to laser surgery, but it may cause skin discoloration in dark-skinned individuals and is usually ineffective against keloids.

Chemical peel. Chemo-exfoliation uses a mild acid preparation to remove superficial scar tissue.

Collagen injections. For depressed scars that are well below the surface of surrounding skin, collagen injections may be used to build up the scar tissue. The body responds to the injections by sending in fibrin to establish its own growth network. Within six weeks to three months, the collagen is absorbed, leaving the new connective tissue well established. Unfortunately, allergic reactions may occur, and the process must be repeated every six months to two years, since the collagen results are only temporary.

Silicone treatment. This method, though not approved by the U.S. Food and Drug Administration (FDA) for medical use, is also used to fill depressed scars; however, it carries additional risks such as a tendency to migrate.

Fibrel injections. This new substance has been tested as an alternative to collagen in a national multicenter study in the United States. Made from a sample of the person's own blood, taken during an office visit, a small amount of plasma is mixed with a gelatin base and an anticlotting agent and injected. So far, results are promising. "Fibrel has lasted up to a year in our one-year follow-up study," says Ivan Cohen, M.D., a Fairfield, Connecticut, dermatologist, who participated in the study. "Hopefully, it will last even longer." According to Dr. Cohen, none of the 321 patients treated with Fibrel has had a reaction or shown sensitivity. The FDA is completing the approval process and Fibrel should be widely available in the near future.

Plastic surgery. Surgical revision by plastic surgery can greatly improve how a scar looks, but it does not completely remove it. A bad scar may be surgically removed and the skin resutured, with after-care to prevent new scar formation. A very large scar may be treated with a "Z-plasty," which changes the scar's direction, interrupting its line and length. After his burn injury, A. J. had four skin grafts and then two Z-plasties. He says, "I could tell the improvement the Z-plasty made immediately."

Several types of "plasties" can be performed to disguise a scar. In some cases, flaps of skin from normal areas can be used to partially disguise large scars. If body movements cause tension along the scar line, skin grafts may be necessary.

Large keloids, once believed to be inoperable, can be surgically removed, leaving only a small border edge of keloid tissue from the original scar, which is sutured together. New keloid tissue does not regenerate from the old keloid, so the original scar can be greatly reduced.

X-ray therapy. Despite the cancer risk, some physicians

feel there is still a place for carefully monitored x-ray therapy, especially on recalcitrant keloids, which do not have many other revision options. Radiation inhibits scar tissue growth.

New Hope

Promising new scar research continues. Live yeast cell derivatives (LYCD) have been found to enhance wound healing by stimulating the formation of new blood vessels (angiogenesis), increasing oxygen consumption and improving collagen synthesis. A study at the Burn Center of Alta Bates Hospital in Berkeley, California, shows that the LYCD significantly accelerates wound healing. "Results were excellent," says Vicky Balagno, nursing care coordinator. "There was better healing and less scarring." Manufacturers are currently working toward FDA approval.

Electricity may also enhance wound healing. Research has shown that the skin contains "battery potentials" within the epidermis that channel electricity into wounds. The ability to manipulate these currents may provide a means to regenerate injured tissue.

Another avenue of research is hypnosis, which has scientifically demonstrated its ability to promote healing by redirecting blood flow and volume. In one study, burn patients were able to direct blood flow to one side of the body by imagery and suggestion, accelerating their rate of healing.

While researchers arc far from solving all the mysteries of scar formation, new information and prevention techniques offer new hope that being "scarred for life" may someday be a thing of the past.

PART VI: MEN'S HEALTH NEWSFRONT

CHAPTER 27

New Help for Sexual Problems

When the spirit is willing but the body isn't able, the latest advice and newest devices from the medical profession may be able to help.

Some deal with it by slipping into the library for self-help manuals. Braver souls schedule a doctor's appointment "for a . . . uh, um, . . . problem." Many merely muffle sad sighs into the pillow, night after night.

As one man put it, "Sexual problems have got to be *the* hardest thing in the world to talk about with anyone."

Sexual dysfunction is at least becoming less difficult to treat, if not to discuss. The fields of sexual medicine and psychosexual therapy are yielding answers to the distressing but not uncommon question, "Why can't I make love?"

When the Body Won't

Nearly ten million American men share the problem of impotence, a condition sort of like a started car with four flat tires that can't go anywhere. It's a matter of faulty mechanics: Impotent men may *desire* sex, but their bodies are unable to achieve and maintain erections capable of vaginal penetration.

Almost every man goes through some *brief* period of impotence at least once in his life. This is probably normal and could just be the result of not enough sleep, too many financial or career worries, or other stress.

"A few weeks of this temporary impotence is nothing to worry about," says Jack Jaffe, M.D., medical director of the Potency Recovery Center in Los Angeles (Panorama City). "When months go by, though, some concern may be in order and a cause should be sought."

The cause might be psychogenic, calling for counseling to explore why the mind has put up a roadblock to sex. Fear of impregnating a woman or a trigger event such as an extramarital affair are only two of the many explanations physicians discover. "Doctor, I was fine until about two weeks ago . . . " is one clue that the impotence is psychologically rooted.

But in roughly 30 to 50 percent of all impotency cases, the trouble is organic, or physical, in nature. "A tip-off to organic impotency is if the patient says, 'I can't figure it out—it just sort of eased up on me and got gradually worse,' " explains Michael Pfeifer, M.D., an endocrinologist and associate professor of medicine at the University of Louisville School of Medicine.

Diabetes, atherosclerosis, high blood pressure and other medical conditions are frequently to blame. (As many as half of all diabetic men become impotent.) In addition to the illnesses themselves, the medications used to treat them often invite impotence.

To first determine if the impotence is of a psychogenic or organic nature, doctors study penis activity during REM sleep, the stage where dreams and (usually) multiple erections take place.

"Blood flow increases in REM sleep and swells the penis," Dr. Pfeifer says. (The equivalent of this in females is a vaginal flush.) "But if a medical problem interferes with blood flow, the penis will stay flaccid. The oldest method to monitor REM activity used a strip of postage stamps wrapped around the shaft. In the morning, if the perforations were broken, we could assume an erection had taken place and the man was physically capable of having intercourse. Therefore we told him, 'You're normal; the problem is with your mind or your desire.' But what we really were seeing was evidence of tumescence, or soft swelling, and not rigidity, the full hardness needed to make love."

Two monitoring improvements were developed that could tell *where* on the penis—the base, shaft or tip—response was lacking. But with a new robotic-type device, doctors can assess rigidity for the first time. "This is exciting—now we can truly differentiate between psychogenic and organic trouble," says Dr. Pfeifer. The device is called a rigiscan, and it can assess tumescence and rigidity at the base and tip during sleep. It consists of two bands around the penis, with wires that connect to a computer chip attached to the leg. The memory chip can then be played back on an IBM computer in the morning for a truer-than-ever picture of erectile ability.

If two to five nights of REM testing indicate a physical problem, further medical screening can look for hormonal trouble, which shows up in 2 to 4 percent of impotency cases and can usually be successfully treated by an endocrinologist; vascular impairment, which keeps enough blood from getting to the penis in 10 to 30 percent of impotent men and can respond to new, intricate vein and artery surgery; or nerve problems, determined mainly by a diagnosis of exclusion.

When the bottom line is impotence that can't be cured by eliminating the physical condition, technology offers four possible ways to produce erections strong enough for making love. They're listed here from least to most recommended by doctors.

Vasodilators. These are oral medications (yohimbine and nitroglycerin) used with mild success to dilate blood vessels. "This approach is still experimental, and there are better options," Dr. Jaffe notes.

Injections. The drugs papaverine and phentolamine (Regitine) combine in this new concept of self-administered penile shots. Increased blood flow produces the

(continued on page 196)

Erection Injections: "Magic Bullet" for Impotence?

"It's amazing, it really is," says Adrian Zorgniotti, M.D., director of urology at Cabrini Medical Center in New York City. Adds reproductive microsurgeon Sherman Silber, M.D., of St. Luke's West Hospital in St. Louis, "I'm just extraordinarily impressed with how simple it is. It's really going to revolutionize the treatment of impotence."

What these two prominent urologists are talking about is erection-producing injections of a drug called papaverine, combined with a second drug, an obscure alpha-blocker called phentolamine (Regitine).

"We've found that 76 percent of the impotent men we've treated can successfully have sex after the injections, regardless of their age or the etiology [cause] of their problem," says Dr. Zorgniotti, who was the first to use the new drug combination. "And I'm not talking about running it 5 percent up the flagpole—I'm talking about a complete reversal of the problem." Even men whose impotence is caused by diabetes, neurologic problems, heart disease or radical cancer surgery may respond to the shots, Dr. Zorgniotti says, adding that "I've actually helped three patients consummate their marriages."

Dr. Silber reports that among his patients, the success rate is also around 80 percent and that "*everybody* gets at least a minor erection." The new treatment is so far superior to the old injections that neither doctor is even using papaverine alone anymore.

Who *doesn't* respond to the injections? Usually, men over the age of 70 or those who are seriously ill, very often with advanced heart disease, Dr. Zorgniotti says.

Naturally, there's a down side to this story. The main drawback is that you have to give yourself these injections directly into the penis every time the mood strikes. "It could never be an effective treatment unless we taught men to inject themselves," Dr. Silber says. And though he insists that "it's painless; I guarantee it," lots of men may find it hard to envision slipping even a tiny needle into that most private of all possessions. (Dr. Zorgniotti says he's currently working on the idea of a permanently implanted, drug-filled bulb that would produce an erection with a couple of deft squeezes. But that development is still years away.)

On the other hand, Dr. Silber reports, about 20 percent of the time, five or six initial shots effect a "permanent cure," fully restoring erectile function without any further injections. "It's my suspicion that in these cases, the shots are just unmasking psychogenic [psychologically caused] impotence," he says. "But so what? It works better than therapy."

Another drawback is cost. Regitine is an expensive drug—about eight times as expensive as papaverine. In fact, Dr. Zorgniotti charges a flat fee of $2,400 a year for patients using the injections (that's good for ten shots a month). This cost is often partially reimbursed by medical insurance.

And although so far no serious side effects have turned up, it's possible that regular injections eventually may cause problems. The most troubling possibility so far is that, in some men, fibrous changes in the penis have developed after repeated injections. This may be a previously undiagnosed but unrelated problem (Peyronie's disease) or a long-term consequence of the treatment. But "I see no intelligent reason to suspect long-term problems," Dr. Silber says.

(continued)

Erection Injections—*Continued*

Also, in about 6 percent of patients, the solution becomes the problem: These robust new erections won't go away. They're easily deflated with injections of another drug called norepinephrine. Still, it's a possibility with an uncomfortably high potential for comic melodrama.

If all those drawbacks are not enough to dissuade you, you may be a candidate for injections.

fullest, most natural-looking erection of any artificial aid and will last 30 to 120 minutes.

Suction devices. Resembling either condoms or cylinders, the two new suction methods create a vacuum to make an erection that will last about a half hour. "This might be a good method if you don't want one of the other approaches and can't undergo surgery for an implant," says Dr. Pfeifer, "but there are minuses: The penis gets stiff but not really hard. Sperm are blocked by the rubber band used to keep blood in the penis, and fathering children can't happen. [It's not to be used as a birth control method, though.] And there's extreme danger to the organ if the man falls asleep and doesn't take off the rubber band."

Prostheses. Penile implants get the highest marks from physicians and from most of the 350,000 men in America who have them. Seventeen studies by 25 urologists indicate over 90 percent of the men and women whose sex lives depend upon a prosthesis accept it and are emotionally satisfied with the results.

Although the idea of penile implants is not new (men have been getting them for more than 20 years), there have been tremendous improvements in design and function.

In Dr. Pfeifer's opinion, "An implant carries less risk than other impotence treatments, is more romantic because it allows spontaneity, lets the man father children and gives a better-quality sex life."

There are several styles of implants to choose from. One is the semirigid type. During simple, inexpensive surgery, two flexible rods are implanted in the penis that allow a man to bend it up for intercourse and down close to the body when not in use. "There are no parts to break down with this version," says Dr. Jaffe, "but the man is still somewhat stiff and elongated when not making love."

Another implant is inflatable. Balloon-shaped implant material makes a penis with this aid look more natural when erect and truly flaccid afterward. The man pumps an implanted reservoir to harden (it takes effort to inflate) and can achieve large, full-girth erections. "This method seems to give the highest satisfaction to couples," notes Dr. Pfeifer. The drawbacks: Many parts are involved and in some cases will need repair in one to five years. Also, the implant requires longer, more invasive surgery and is more expensive.

The self-contained type of implant also uses the pump concept, but it is combined with rods. It has fewer parts than the inflatable one and is less complicated to install. The penis with a self-contained implant will look only semiflaccid when not erect, "a potential problem for men who shower in a gym after a workout or similar social situation," Dr. Pfeifer says.

A fourth prosthesis will be available soon; it consists of a ball, socket and rod-type design and "works like clicking a ballpoint pen to become erect and then flaccid," explains Dr. Pfeifer. The appearance of the penis will be neither fully erect nor totally flaccid.

One prosthesis isn't necessarily better than the others, and a doctor should explain in detail each type of implant available, along with their advantages and shortcomings. Picking a prosthesis is basically a matter of lifestyle.

"One 72-year-old man I treated enjoys close ballroom dancing every weekend," says Dr. Jaffe. "He wanted the one that would feel the most natural, chose a pump type, and put up with the hassle of inflating because of what was important in his life."

The end result of impotence treatment—a restored sex

life—is a tremendous relief to both the man and woman who have had to deal with the dilemma. "I've gotten more Christmas cards from former impotency patients than I did in over 20 years of treating cancer patients," notes Dr. Jaffe.

How Satisfying Are Penile Implants?

Surgical implantation of a pair of inflatable rods directly into the penis is an increasingly common solution to chronic, long-term impotence.

How do the recipients of these devices feel about them after months or years of use? "The long-term emotional results vary from sheer delight to frustration, disappointment and outright dislike for the implant," says Fletcher C. Derrick, M.D., clinical professor of urology at the Medical University of South Carolina, Charleston.

In his experience, 85 to 90 percent of patients are very happy with the implant, about 10 percent are somewhat disappointed, and 2 to 5 percent are totally unhappy.

Those who are most gratified, he says, are men who have some sensation in their genitals and at least some erectile capacity left. Those who have had long-term impotence and little or no sensation are likely to be disappointed, Dr. Derrick says, because "an implant does not provide a return of normal sensation and climax." Also, he adds, "implants almost never achieve the patient's idea of size."

Still, he says, not one of his patients, even those who've expressed the greatest disappointment, has requested that his implant be removed (*Medical Aspects of Human Sexuality*).

A Problem of Timing

Premature ejaculation can trouble a couple's sex life just as impotence can. With this problem, a man's orgasm catches him off guard; he isn't aware that he is about to climax until it starts happening. When this situation becomes chronic, self-help or sexual therapy may enable the man to regain control.

The old school of psychosexual thought considered distraction to be the most effective weapon for combating premature ejaculation. The man should get his mind off his arousal, either by counting backward or thinking about baseball or something equally distracting, in order to let an impending orgasm subside and so prolong intercourse. This never really worked, and the updated approach stresses the opposite behavior.

"To increase control, a man must pay particular attention to the sensation in his body as he becomes more and more aroused," says Georgia Witkin-Lanoil, Ph.D., in her book *The Male Stress Syndrome*. The goal is to recognize premonitory sensations, the body signals that herald the first phase of orgasm, the emission phase. This is when semen arrives in the urethra; ejaculation is only a few seconds away.

If a man tunes in and learns these sensations, "he can slow his thrusting, alter the type of stimulation he is receiving, change position or even pause until control is regained," explains Dr. Witkin-Lanoil, who teaches in the psychiatry department of Mount Sinai Medical College in New York City.

Enjoying and paying extra attention to arousal can prevent surprise orgasms, and there are some ways to learn this. One is the stop/start technique. A man can stimulate himself until orgasmic sensations begin to build and then stop all movement until the urgency fades. Three cycles of starting and stopping can be followed by an ejaculation. When this is mastered, four, five and six cycles can be practiced, and then repeated in the same manner with a partner.

Another method is the squeeze technique. This involves both partners and a similar cycle theory. "When the man feels his orgasm building, his partner can stop it by firmly squeezing the penis at the base of the tip with her thumb and forefingers," explains sex therapist Bob Kinder, Ph.D., associate professor of psychology in the clinical and health psychology doctoral program at the University of South Florida. Dr. Kinder notes couples have over a 90 percent success rate when they use these methods to overcome premature ejaculation.

CHAPTER 28

Why Men Are Afraid of Doctors

A multitude of macho mandates keeps many men from getting the health care they need.

Lurking in a dark, unexplored corner of the male brain is a tiny but insidious fear. Even the burliest of men are afraid of doctors.

It gets them young—as early as the age of eight, say school nurses—and grows with the years, until the very sight of a white jacket can start a grown man's knees knocking.

Well, perhaps it's not as bad as all that, but it is a fact that American men visit doctors' offices 20 percent less than women, while their mortality rates are slightly higher. Many experts say that, among the reasons keeping men away from health-care professionals, fear ranks high.

"I surveyed men while writing my book and asked them what they are most afraid of," says Georgia Witkin-Lanoil, Ph.D., a lecturer in the Department of Psychiatry at Mount

Sinai Medical College in New York City and author of *The Male Stress Syndrome.* "Doctors of all kinds scored very high," she says. She also found that men are more afraid of illness than of death.

"Men are afraid of doctors," says Francis Baumli, Ph.D., a medical health consultant in Columbia, Missouri, and a representative of the Coalition of Free Men, a national men's rights organization. "A man going to see a doctor is walking into an entirely foreign environment. He has to take his clothes off in front of a perfect stranger. A man has to have his body touched in areas where he would probably never touch himself, where his wife may not even touch him during lovemaking."

This type of fear stems, in part, from men's unfamiliarity with their own bodies.

"Men are conditioned from the time they are little boys not to be in touch with their bodies," explains Dr. Baumli. "It's much less okay for a little boy to complain to his mother or father of pain than for a little girl."

At puberty, girls get lots of helpful hints from their mothers and teachers, but boys are left virtually in the dark. "Fathers rarely sit down and say, 'Hey son, something wonderful is about to happen to you. You're going to grow hair on your body and get pimples, and you're going to be filled with strange desires you won't understand,'' says Sherman Silber, M.D., a reproductive microsurgeon at St. Luke's West Hospital in St. Louis and author of *The Male*.

All this alienation of the male psyche from the male body leads to men being extremely nervous when their bodies become the center of attention, which is just what happens when they go to doctors. But that is only a problem if they actually make it into the doctor's office. Their discomfort and lack of knowledge of their bodies can make that a rare occasion indeed.

That's partially because men often don't realize they have any need for a doctor. "Men are absolutely unaware of the most blatant body signals," says Dr. Baumli. "Their perceptive faculties have been so numbed by the masculinizing factors of our society that their bodies could be screaming to them for help and they wouldn't notice."

Sometimes a man's lack of familiarity with his own body can have disastrous results. "A high school teacher, about 40 years old, had walked around with a very bad pain in his chest for a week," says Dr. Baumli. "He had mentioned it to a couple of people and said that he thought he had pulled a muscle. The man dropped dead of a heart attack a week later."

Even when they do realize they need to see a physician, many men avoid the inevitable because the doctors themselves make their male patients just plain uneasy. "Women are brought into contact with the medical profession far more frequently than men in this society," explains Constance Nathanson, Ph.D., of the School of Hygiene and Public Health at Johns Hopkins University. Many aspects of women's lives, such as menstruation, childbearing and the care of families, bring them to doctors regularly and allow them to become comfortable with the medical profession in a way that most men never experience.

The Strong, Silent Type

Besides simply not being used to doctors, men have other reasons to fear seeking medical help. Our culture says that men must be strong and invulnerable; men who are not can face ridicule and scorn from their peers. "It's not macho to recognize that you need a doctor," says Dr. Nathanson. "Help-seeking is traditionally seen as a kind of female thing."

And complaining of pain is seen as a weakness. "My dad lived with a pain in his belly for a couple of weeks without saying anything about it," relates Laurel DenHartog, information coordinator of the United Cancer Council. "When he finally said something, we rushed him to the hospital, and it turned out that he'd been walking around with a ruptured appendix and a bellyful of peritonitis. He had to have emergency surgery, all because it's not manly to complain."

Being macho means, for many men, not ever feeling ill. It also can mean always being independent and in control.

"The sick role is a dependent one, which men may be reluctant to take on," says John Wheat, M.D., M.P.H., who is associated with the University of Tennessee at Memphis.

Dr. Witkin-Lanoil, too, believes that men avoid doctors because they fear appearing, or even becoming, vulnerable or dependent. "Going to a doctor, for men, is putting themselves in someone else's hands," she says. "This is very frightening for men because they are trained to maintain control over every aspect of their lives."

The illnesses men get as a result of stress, such as high blood pressure, can really put them on the spot. "If men are told they have become ill as a result of stress, they feel guilt," says Dr. Witkin-Lanoil. "They interpret the situation as meaning they should have kept better control, when in fact, the truth is just the opposite. They should have given up control and allowed themselves to be vulnerable."

Yet giving up this facade of invulnerability is very difficult for men. "Lots of men, from the president of a large company to a policeman, told me change is frightening to them," says Dr. Witkin-Lanoil. "When a man goes to a doctor, very much of what he fears is that he's going to be told to change his lifestyle."

The changes they fear could be as simple as having to exercise more to avoid high blood pressure or as terrifying as being hospitalized or operated on for a serious illness.

The fear of being told they are very sick often keeps men from doctors. "Sometimes gay men come down with a sore throat and are afraid to go to a doctor because they think it might be AIDS," says Kenneth Solomon, M.D., an adjunct assistant professor of psychiatry at the University of Maryland and a staff psychiatrist at the Sheppard and Enoch Pratt Hospital in Baltimore.

"Fear can be part of men's reactions, particularly when you're talking about prostate or testicular cancer," says Laurel DenHartog. Yet, she says, the treatment for these kinds of cancer does not necessarily cause the emasculation many men fear. The cancer itself could mean death, however, if it is not caught early enough. "Where cancer is concerned, early detection is the key," she emphasizes.

Fear often stems from ignorance, and Dr. Silber says that men rarely do the kind of research on their bodies that women do regularly. This can make some men embarrassingly squeamish. "Before doing certain procedures, we usually show patients a video of the operation to help alleviate their anxiety," says Dr. Silber. "Many men want to watch it, and many do," he continues. "But lots say they'd rather not watch it, and some actually faint while it's going on. All of the women watch it," he adds.

Some people say that women are more comfortable with doctors and go to doctors more than men simply because they have more illnesses. That idea, however, doesn't hold much water. "Many of women's routine, healthy experiences have been medicalized," explains Catherine Kohler Riessman, Ph.D., a professor of sociology and social work at Smith College. These routine experiences—childbearing, contraception and what Dr. Riessman calls the "medical beauty industry," which provides cosmetic surgery and weight-loss drugs—take women to doctors on a far more frequent basis than men. "It is interesting to note," she says, "that men's routine experiences—balding, for instance—have not been medicalized in the same way."

Facing Up to Fear

How can men overcome their fears and start taking advantage of the help doctors are there to give? Laurel DenHartog says a reeducation of male thought processes is necessary. "They have to realize that putting off medical treatment is not intelligent; it is not manly. It is stupid," she says.

Basically, men have to convince themselves that it is more helpful to them to see a doctor regularly than to protect their macho image or avoid finding out that they are ill. "When they see the risk:reward ratio—let's put this into male language—they'll see the risk of not getting care is much higher than the risk of losing control or changing their lifestyle," says Dr. Witkin-Lanoil. "And the reward of taking care of themselves is much higher than the reward of kidding themselves that nothing is wrong for a few months until it gets too bad to ignore."

One way to feel more in control when seeing a physician is to approach the situation as an educated consumer. "You are entitled to shop for a doctor," says Dr. Witkin-Lanoil. "And you are entitled to have a physician you can relate to and talk to, whom you can respect."

Yet sometimes a man's fear of appearing vulnerable makes it impossible to be open with the doctor in return. "Men are taught that other men may use weaknesses against them," explains Dr. Witkin-Lanoil. Her advice to men who feel this way is to see a female doctor. "Female doctors are seen as more nurturing and less of a threat," she says. "It may be easier for a man to seek help from a woman than another man."

Before the problem of *which* doctor to see, however, is the problem of knowing *when* to see a doctor. To become better at this, men must get more in touch with their bodies. "Men have to re-create the learning process they didn't have as children," says Dr. Silber. "If they do, their health will improve. They will become more aware of watching their weight, they'll get into exercise, and they'll learn to reduce stress."

One of the easiest ways to get in touch with your body is simply to relax and let yourself go. Set aside a part of the day to do nothing—really nothing, not watching TV with a newspaper in front of you—says Dr. Baumli, and you'll suddenly become much more aware of how your body feels. "A man who never slows down enough to hear the ticking of his own heart is never going to have the chance to find out if his body is ill," he says.

Men just have to learn to pay attention to their health more than to their fears. But it is difficult. Lots of times, doctors are no better at this than anyone else. The last time Dr. Solomon was sick, he says, he self-diagnosed himself as probably having pneumonia, rather than going to a doctor. He decided to treat himself with penicillin and got slightly better. So then, still ill and still not having seen a doctor, he went off to New Orleans and had fun for five days. "That's the way you treat these problems, right?" he jokes.

By the time he returned from his trip, he had been sick for two months, with few signs of improvement. "Finally my girlfriend made it clear that if I wanted to hang around her, I'd better go to a doctor," he says. "I did, the doctor said I had bronchitis, gave me a different antibiotic, and I was better in two days."

So take heart, men. And take yourselves to the doctor when you really ought to go.

CHAPTER 29

Fighting Back against Prostate Trouble

Among men, 11 percent have never heard of this troublesome gland. Half don't even recognize prostate symptoms. Yet virtually all men experience problems.

The prostate gland produces most of the fluid in semen, but it's best known for causing problems. Please note: There is no "r" in the name of this pesky gland. It's *prostate*, not *prostrate*. Prostrate means lying face-down, a posture many urologists are tempted to assume after years of hearing the word mispronounced.

Most men develop at least one of the four most common prostate problems by age 60, yet a survey showed that 11 percent of American men have never heard of the gland, and 57 percent have no idea what symptoms prostate problems might cause. Most women know even less about this mysterious doughnut-shaped gland, situated below the male bladder about two inches above the rectum.

The prostate is not a single gland but rather a collection of 30 to 50 small, gland-cell clusters, organized into several lobes held together by fibrous connective tissue. If the prostate as a whole resembles a doughnut, then the urethra, the tube through which urine and semen pass, runs through the doughnut hole. A valve allows urine—but not semen—to flow when the penis is flaccid. When the penis is erect, the valve blocks urine but allows semen to flow. The prostate is almond-size in young boys, but during puberty, the male sex hormone testosterone stimulates it to mature to the size of a large walnut, and it begins to produce seminal fluid. Unlike other glands, the prostate continues to grow with age. In some men it can reach the size of a grapefruit. But around age 50, prostate overgrowth (hypertrophy) causes noticeable problems in about 20 percent of men. By age 70, that figure rises to more than 50 percent.

Until recently, three conditions were believed to account for the vast majority of prostate problems: inflammation (bacterial prostatitis), noncancerous overgrowth (benign hypertrophy) and prostate cancer. Recently, however, for reasons explained below, urologists have been reconsidering prostatitis, and the emerging consensus is that much of what was once called bacterial prostatitis may involve nonbacterial microorganisms or no germs at all. Nonbacterial prostatitis is a relatively new concept, and urologists have not settled on a name for the condition. It is variously known as "prostatosis," "prostatodynia" and "urinary sphincter hypertonicity" (USH).

Prostatitis

Before the new varieties of this illness were delineated, bacterial prostatitis was considered the most common urologic problem in men under 50. Symptoms were said to include fever; pain in the penis, lower abdomen, lower back or perineum (the area between the scrotum and the anus); pain or burning on urination and/or ejaculation; and "voiding dysfunction" (an urgent need to urinate frequently, scant urine production, trouble starting urination and "nocturia," the need to urinate frequently at night).

Prostatitis was assumed to be caused by either gonorrhea or the *Escherichia coli* bacteria responsible for urinary tract infections in women. But oddly, prostatitis symptoms varied tremendously, bacteria could be cultured only rarely, and it was transmitted sexually to women much less frequently than other bacterial infections, such as gonorrhea, for example.

The reason for this was that the microorganisms responsible for prostatitis were not always *Escherichia coli* but sometimes *Chlamydia, Mycoplasma* or *Trichomonas,* which did not grow in the culture media urologists used. "*Mycoplasma* may cause the majority of prostatitis," says John Owen Marks, M.D., a New York City urologist affiliated with Beth Israel Hospital. Recently, two relatively simple tests for *Chlamydia* have become available, and most urologists now culture prostatic fluid for this bacterialike organism. In cases of chronic inflammation, Dr. Marks suggests that men also request workups for *Mycoplasma* and *Trichomonas.*

If a man has voiding dysfunction and pain, but no fever, no identifiable microorganisms and no unusually large number of white blood cells, an index of infection, the current thinking is that he does not have bacterial prostatitis but this new, unnamed condition, currently a focus of considerable controversy among urologists.

"Prostatosis and prostatodynia are catchall diagnoses that mean we don't know what's causing the problem," Dr. Marks says. "In such cases I try a variety of antibiotics and recommend hot baths, changes in sexual activity and elimination of alcohol—especially red wine—strong teas, spicy foods and coffee—both caffeinated and decaffeinated—any of which may irritate the prostate."

"Prostatodynia is a garbage diagnosis," counters Ira Sharlip, M.D., an assistant clinical professor of urology at the University of California's San Francisco Medical Center. "All it means is 'pain in the prostate.' In the absence of identifiable microorganisms and elevated white cells, I believe that most prostatitis is actually USH, stress-related tension in the muscle that controls urination. The man is uptight, and so is his urinary sphincter. In my opinion, prostatitis has been seriously overdiagnosed, and although some prostatitis may be caused by *Chlamydia* or other organisms, most of these cases involve muscle tension. We rarely find microorganisms and white cells in men whose symptoms are limited to voiding dysfunction and perineal pain because there are none."

Dr. Sharlip treats USH by explaining its basis in muscle tension and reassuring the man that the condition, though annoying, is medically minor. "A man who experiences pain in the penis or perineum, or pain in ejaculation, can develop morbid fears," Dr. Sharlip says. "Such fears can aggravate stress-related problems. Reassurance that the problem is minor often helps considerably." The problem usually clears up in a week or so with hot baths, stress-management techniques and, in some cases, a prescription muscle relaxant (Minipress).

Dr. Marks agrees that some nonbacterial prostatitis may be caused by stress, which is why he recommends hot baths, but he urges men not to accept a diagnosis of "stress" unless workups for *Chlamydia, Mycoplasma* and *Trichomonas* have turned out negative.

There are two kinds of prostatitis, acute and chronic. The former causes sudden fever and genital, abdominal and/or low back pain. (The prostate is located near the base of the back.) Acute prostatitis usually clears up in about a week with the sulfa-based antibiotic trimethoprim/sulfamehoxazole (Bactrim, Septra). Chronic prostatitis, which may or may not be caused by a microorganism, causes less severe symptoms but lasts longer. It may require more lab work, longer-term antibiotics, stress management and the dietary modifications described above.

"Chronic prostatitis," Dr. Sharlip says, "often turns out to be nothing more than persistent USH. But if the gland feels inflamed, I prescribe antibiotics, and it often helps to eliminate caffeine and alcohol."

Prostatitis was once thought to be associated with sexual abstinence ("priests' disease") or irregular or binging sexual activity ("sailors' disease"—after months of presumed abstinence at sea, some sailors developed prostatitis after sexual binges ashore). Today these observations seem naive. Many men who abstain from sex never develop prostatitis. There is no evidence that sailors abstain, then binge; masturbation is certainly available at sea. And many extremely sexually active men never develop this illness, Dr. Sharlip says. "The studies I've seen do not support either sexual irregularity or sexual binging as risk factors for prostatitis."

Sexual abstinence, however, may contribute to USH. For many men, sex is a key means—for some, the only means—of stress management. Without reasonably regular sexual release, some men may focus their stress burdens below the belt.

What about sex during episodes of prostatitis or USH? "Some urologists recommend regular ejaculation," Dr. Sharlip says. "Others recommend temporary abstinence to rest the prostate. I advise men to do what feels most comfortable for them. But if a man experiences pain on ejaculation, he'll probably want to abstain for a while."

Bacterial prostatitis is usually an uncomplicated illness, but if an infected prostate clamps down on the urethra and prevents the bladder from emptying completely, the infection may spread to the bladder (cystitis). The symptoms of cystitis and prostatitis can be quite similar—pain and/or burning on urination and urinary urgency and hesitancy with scant production. But with cystitis, a urinalysis shows the presence of bacteria. Men with chronic bacterial prostatitis should request urinalysis if their physician does not. Like prostatitis, cystitis is not a major medical problem, but if left untreated, it may progress to a kidney infection, which is considerably more serious and often requires hospitalization.

Prostatitis does not predispose a man to prostate cancer. In men over 50, however, it might be a symptom of bladder cancer. "Some physicians keep treating what they think is chronic prostatitis," says James Smolev, M.D., an assistant professor of urology at Johns Hopkins University School of Medicine, "only to discover too late that the man has a bladder tumor. Physicians need to be more thorough when men over 50 come in with prostatitis."

Benign Prostatic Hypertrophy (BPH)

A 20-year-old's prostate is about the size of a walnut, but by age 50 it may have grown much larger. This growth is not cancer, nor does it predispose a man to cancer. It may, however, pinch the urethra and cause urinary urgency, hesitancy and particularly the need to get up at night. Eventually, the man may grow tired of the inconvenience and opt for surgical correction, typically a transurethral resection of the prostate (TURP). With the man under spinal or general anesthesia, the urologist inserts a tiny instrument (resectoscope) into the urethra. When electrically heated, the wire loop at the end of the resectoscope burns away prostatic overgrowth (electrocautery) and widens the urethral path. TURPs are considered routine; nonetheless, they're major surgery. Recovery usually involves three to five days of hospitalization and a week of rest at home. Although surgical complications are uncommon, several are possible: infection (1 percent risk), bleeding that requires transfusion (1 percent), urinary sphincter damage that causes incontinence (1 percent), and erection impairment (1 to 5 percent).

"TURP-related erection problems," Dr. Sharlip says, "are psychological in origin. There is no physiological reason why this operation, when performed properly, should damage the nerves that control erection."

In most cases, however, TURPs result in "dry orgasm." Scarring from the electrocautery usually closes the ejaculatory ducts, thus blocking the flow of seminal fluid. After a TURP, orgasm feels as pleasurable as ever, but the man does not ejaculate. If seminal fluid still flows at all, it is released backward into the bladder. Backward ejaculation, called retroejaculation, may sound strange, but it's of no medical concern. Any semen mixes with the urine and passes out during urination. No ejaculation means no vehicle for sperm to leave the penis. The testicles continue to produce sperm, but they are reabsorbed by the body. Although TURP signals the end of male fertility, this is rarely a problem because the operation is typically performed on men who don't plan to father any more children. Sometimes, however, a man must choose between BPH symptoms and fertility, in which case sperm banking might be an alternative.

Although surgery continues to be the treatment of choice for BPH, the blood pressure drug phenoxybenzamine (Dibenzyline) has produced some intriguing results. In a ten-year study of 171 Israeli men, Dr. Marco Caine of Hadassah Medical Center in Jerusalem reports that 80 percent experienced subjective improvement and 46 percent experienced a doubling of urine flow with a daily dose of ten milligrams of the drug. Unfortunately, phenoxybenzamine is mutagenic in rodents and may be carcinogenic in humans. At this writing, the treatment remains experimental, and few U.S. urologists use it.

Prostate Cancer

Prostate cancer is extremely common—some say almost inevitable—in older men. On autopsy, cancerous cells are found in 10 percent of men in their fifties, one-third of those in their sixties and more than three-quarters of those over 80. Fortunately, most prostate tumors are slow growing, never spread beyond the gland itself, do not cause symptoms and pose no threat to life. "Most men die with prostate cancer, not from it," Dr. Sharlip says.

On the other hand, fast-spreading prostate cancer is the number two cause of cancer death in men. (Lung cancer is number one.) Most common in men over 40, it accounts for 19 percent of men's cancers and 10 percent of male cancer deaths.

The tragedy is that many of these deaths could be prevented with earlier detection, which is relatively simple with the digital rectal exam (DRE). To perform DRE, the physician inserts a gloved finger into the rectum and feels (palpates) the prostate. If any hard lumps are detected, a biopsy is performed. Unfortunately, many physicians do not perform this exam routinely, and men over 40 rarely request it. Gerald Murphy, M.D., professor of urology at the State University of New York at Buffalo, estimates that one-third of men over 40 have never had a DRE, and two-thirds have not had one in the past year. As a result, 60 percent of prostate cancer is diagnosed only after significant symptoms or metastases have developed—and the death rate remains high.

Prostate exams are recommended annually for men over 40. Any biopsy that shows cancer also reveals whether it's slow growing and not particularly dangerous or fast growing and likely to spread. For slow-growing cancers, most urologists advise no treatment, just exams once or twice a year.

Early prostate cancer symptoms include blood in the urine, urinary urgency and hesitancy with scant production and possibly pain. Fast-growing prostate cancer is diagnosed before it has spread beyond the gland only about 20 percent of the time. In such cases, treatment choices include radiation or prostate removal (radical prostatectomy). Radical prostatectomy, which involves either an abdominal or perineal incision, has long been the more popular approach. Until recently, however, it left 90 percent of men nonerective because the nerves that control erection run along the gland and were severed to remove it. Radiation causes nonerection less frequently (about 50 percent of the time), but has other side effects: diarrhea, bowel problems, urethral obstruction and blood in the urine.

Today, however, prostatectomy need not cause erection impairment. Patrick Walsh, M.D., director of the Brady Urological Institute at Johns Hopkins University, has developed a new technique for radical prostatectomy that preserves erection in about 80 percent of cases. "I always wondered why about 10 percent of men could still have erections after radical prostatectomy. It seemed logical to assume that their erectile nerves somehow remained uninjured during surgery. The problem was that despite all we know about anatomy, we didn't know the precise pathways of these nerves around the prostate. In some cases, the surgeon just got lucky and left the nerves intact." Working with a Dutch anatomist, Dr. Walsh mapped the erectile nerves and developed his nerve-sparing prostatectomy technique. It is now available at most major medical centers and should become more widely available as more urologists learn to perform it.

Even if prostate cancer spreads beyond the gland, it is still quite treatable, and survival rates are high. The spread of prostate cancer depends on testosterone. Deprived of the male hormone, most prostate cancers go into dramatic remission.

"When prostate cancer metastasizes," Dr. Sharlip explains, "it often invades the bones, where it causes terrible pain. But once testosterone has been eliminated, I've seen men experience sudden, almost miraculous improvement and live many more years."

But such miracles have a high price. The testicles, which manufacture most of the body's testosterone, must be either removed surgically (castration) or hormonally disabled with estrogen, usually diethylstilbestrol (DES). Either way, the results include erection loss, decreased body hair and possibly breast development and breast pain. (Breast effects can be prevented with radiation.) Currently, researchers are investigating several new chemical treatments for metastatic prostate cancer. All appear to have sexual side effects similar to surgery and DES, but some do not stimulate as much breast development.

Can Zinc Protect the Prostate?

In recent years, nutritionally inclined practitioners have touted zinc as a possible preventive for the entire range of prostate ills. Zinc is an essential trace mineral found in milk, whole grains, peas, carrots and particularly in oysters, long considered a "virility food" in the folk wisdom of several cultures. The prostate has the male body's highest concentration of zinc, and men with prostate problems often show abnormally low zinc levels. Some studies point to preventive and therapeutic possibilities. Others do not. The role of zinc in prostate health remains controversial, though everyone should consume the Recommended Dietary Allowance (RDA), since zinc is an essential mineral.

"I know of no good data showing that zinc prevents or cures prostate problems," Dr. Sharlip says. "But a zinc-rich diet doesn't do any harm."

The same cannot be said, however, for overuse of commercial zinc supplements. The RDA for zinc is 15 milligrams. A dose of 30 milligrams per day is considered quite safe for adults. Symptoms of toxicity—nausea, vomiting, diarrhea and stomach pain—rarely develop unless a man takes 100 to 150 milligrams per day for several weeks. (Zinc also competes with copper. Long-term high doses of zinc may lead to copper deficiency.) Despite the popularity of mineral supplements, most nutritionists recommend obtaining zinc from food sources.

PART VII: WOMEN'S HEALTH NEWSFRONT

CHAPTER 30
Do You Have Osteoporosis?

Knowing the risk factors for this bone-thinning disease is the first step toward a body that will stand up (straight) over time.

You lock your doors, buy a smoke detector and perhaps install a security system to protect the valuables in your home. Do you give the same protection to the valuable strength in your bones?

As a woman, you may be in greater need than men of prevention against osteoporosis, a disease that gradually steals strength-building calcium from your bones. To get an idea whether you'll be standing tall in years to come or whether you'll be one of the millions for whom even a simple task could be backbreaking, see if any of the following risk factors of osteoporosis fit you.

Advancing age means bone strength retreats. It usually isn't until after age 50 or so that neglected bones start demanding attention—usually by fracturing or shortening your stature. Menopause occurs around this time, taking the biggest toll of all on the skeletal system. The diet of an older person is often too poor to maintain bone integrity. And with increasing age, the intestines become less efficient at absorbing what calcium there is in the diet. By the year 2050, it is expected that 22 percent of the U.S. population will be over age 65, making osteoporosis one of the medical profession's top research priorities.

If you're a woman, you must be concerned about your bones. While both sexes unavoidably lose some bone mass simply due to aging, most of the 15 to 20 million cases of advanced osteoporosis are in women. The fact that women have smaller frames than men may be one explanation for the inequity—when the body needs calcium elsewhere and calls on bones to give up part of their supply, men's bones simply have more on reserve.

Menopause, either natural or surgical, means increased risk. Estrogen, the multitalented hormone produced by a woman's ovaries, helps maintain bone mass and strength in addition to its sex-related duties. When menopause shuts down the supply, bones are more susceptible to fractures. Scientists confirmed this estrogen/bone-strength link when they began seeing premature osteoporosis in premenopausal women who have had their ovaries removed. Hormones may also help account for the female bias in osteoporosis. Testosterone, a male hormone helpful for bone mass, has a more gradual decline in production than estrogen, with its somewhat here-today, gone-tomorrow departure. Women who have spent years taking estrogen-containing birth control pills are thought to enjoy greater protection from osteoporosis, also.

Caucasian and Oriental women are at a greater risk than black women. Large-scale studies have repeatedly shown much higher rates of osteoporosis in fairer-skinned races. Two theories may account for this, says Diane Meier, M.D., codirector of the Osteoporosis and Metabolic Bone Disease Program at Mount Sinai Medical Center, New York City. She has conducted a study of 150 white women and 150 black women, ages 26 to 65, to see if the former have a genetic predisposition to excessive bone loss or if nutritional habits and body composition are the key. "Blacks, at least in the North American population, tend to have higher obesity rates. And obesity is protective against bone loss," Dr. Meier explains. (Very thin people, then, are also at greater risk.) Black people may have larger and denser bone structures, too, which may give them an advantage against osteoporosis.

A diet short on calcium will mean bone loss in the long run. Scientists found women who had a calcium-rich diet in childhood and early adulthood built a bone mass more able to withstand osteoporosis in later years. Lactose, a carbohydrate in calcium-laden milk, may help the body absorb calcium. Major health organizations are urging people to start getting the U.S. Recommended Daily Allowance of calcium (800 milligrams for children under the age of four, 1,000 milligrams for adults and children four or more years of age and 1,300 milligrams for pregnant and lactating women) early in life, but most Americans obtain barely half these amounts.

Constant dieters lose more than pounds. They risk losing bone mass, too, after years of passing up high-fat (but also high-calcium) dairy products. Low-fat dairy products like skim milk and cottage cheese can help dieters meet their calcium needs.

Strict vegetarians may restrict their bones' strength. "Pure vegetarians who don't eat any dairy products have a hard time getting adequate calcium," says Dr. Meier. "The green vegetables they eat, like broccoli and spinach, do have calcium, but they also contain oxalates, which block the absorption of calcium in the gut."

A meat-eater's diet may eat away at bone strength. A culinary love affair with red meat puts overindulgers at greater risk—studies indicate high protein levels speed up the excretion of calcium in urine and keep the mineral from making its way to bones.

A vitamin D deficiency could mean low-grade bone strength. Vitamin D is normally obtained in adequate amounts through a healthy diet and through the skin with 10 to 20 minutes of sun exposure daily. It's crucial for intestinal absorption of calcium and bone remodeling. But older people may run into a vitamin D shortage because of poor nutrition and long housebound periods due to illness or injury. The sunshine/vitamin D connection is also why people who live in rainier, cloudier climates are thought to be at higher risk than those on whom the sun always shines.

A family history of osteoporosis is related to your risk of getting the disease. A woman's grandmother, mother and aunt may provide a clue to what may be in store for her. One theory behind this: If female relatives reached menopause at a rather early age, they may pass along that tendency, so more years are spent without estrogen's bone protection.

A lazybones lifestyle leads to thinner bones later. One of the many beneficial effects of exercise on the body is the way it helps build bones. Any weight-bearing exercise stimulates the skeleton to put down new bone. Tennis players, weight lifters, ballet dancers and other athletes show wider bones and more cortical, or outside-layer, bone in limbs involved in their particular sport. And astronauts are prime examples of gravity's usefulness—when they're weightless in space, they lose a significant amount of bone mass. Patients confined to bed face a similar situation and can lose as much as 1 percent of their trabecular, or inner, bone per week. Resuming normal weight-bearing activity gradually restores the bone.

Certain substances make calcium seep away. Prolonged use of aluminum-containing antacids, prednisone- or cortisone-containing drugs and diuretics can increase the risk of bone loss. Excessive sodium in the diet is also being explored as a possible cause of calcium excretion, but this research is still very preliminary.

Medical disorders may be additional risk factors for bone loss. Diabetes, hyperthyroidism, hyperparathyroidism, Cushing's disease, rheumatoid arthritis and gastrectomy have been reported to cause osteoporosis, but scientists note the need for more research in this area.

Cigarette smoking may weaken bones. Smoking is suspected of exerting a possibly toxic effect on bone mass. Women who smoke have lower estrogen levels, tend to be thinner than nonsmokers and undergo menopause at an earlier age. Overall, women smokers appear to have lower cortical bone mass.

Alcohol may abuse bones. Heavy alcohol use is one of

the few things that put a man at risk for osteoporosis. Alcoholic men have lower bone mass and lose bone more rapidly than nonalcoholics. In women, the incidence of hip fractures increases as alcohol intake rises. These associations could stem from a direct toxic effect of alcohol or from poor nutrition, lower body weight, liver disease or other alcohol-related factors.

Making the Risk Factors Less Risky

The medical profession now offers screening clinics, treatment programs and extensive public-education campaigns geared to people at risk. The recommended steps for long-lasting bones are easy for everyone.

Getting adequate calcium and exercise is the best way to build up healthy bone mass and is important for people of all ages, especially those under age 35. Adequate calcium from dairy products, green vegetables, sardines and salmon with edible bones, tofu and other food sources, or from dietary supplements, is essential. Weight-bearing exercise should be done at least five times a week, and it can be anything from walking to tennis.

Be sure to get some sunshine and maintain adequate vitamin D in your diet. Finally, minimize the risk factors in your control, like smoking and alcohol.

Starting the Treatment

With one possible exception, nothing seems to replace bone once it's lost after menopause. Fluoride looks promising for rebuilding bone, but it hasn't been approved by the U.S. Food and Drug Administration (FDA) yet for mass use.

"Women approaching menopause need to consult with their physicians for assessment of diagnosis and should ask about treatment and prevention of the disorder," notes Sandra Raymond, executive director of the National Osteoporosis Foundation in Washington, D.C.

After taking your history and assessing your risk for the disease, doctors at screening clinics can examine the condition of your bones with quick and accurate procedures. If bone seems to be ebbing or your history makes you a likely candidate, you can begin treatment to keep the condition from getting worse.

A boost in calcium is urged by most researchers, even though calcium's postmenopausal role hasn't been documented as well as its effectiveness in building strong bone in childhood and through early adulthood. Doctors suggest 1,000 to 1,500 milligrams of calcium for women at menopause and beyond. This is also about the same amount taken by astronauts after missions.

"If you're taking a supplement," advises Dr. Meier, "take it with juice or fluid independently of meals. Try it first thing in the morning, an hour before breakfast. The juice will stimulate gastric acid for absorption, and delaying breakfast will ensure protein and fiber won't compete with calcium in the gut for absorption."

Walking wins out as the most recommended exercise for postmenopausal women, again done at least five times a week. But the biggest gun in the fight against further bone loss is estrogen supplementation.

The FDA has approved low-dose estrogen to retard further bone loss in postmenopausal women with evidence of loss or deficiency of bone mass. The labeling also states that the estrogen should be used with other measures, such as calcium and exercise. Provided that a woman's health poses no contraindications to estrogen, the therapy seems to be as safe as it is effective.

One study of over 500 women found estrogen users had significantly greater mineral content, fewer wrist and hip fractures and greater cortical thickness than women who didn't receive estrogen. "Long-term estrogen-replacement therapy confers significant protection against bone loss and fracture," the researchers note (*Annals of Internal Medicine*).

Women with either a personal or family history of endometrial or breast cancer probably shouldn't have estrogen therapy, cautions Dr. Meier. "There's a marked increase of

Estrogen May Help Clear Arteries

If you're taking estrogen because menopause is menacing your bones, you may glean an unexpected benefit: protection from coronary artery disease.

A study of more than 900 women who underwent angiography, an x-ray inspection of their blood vessels, found less occlusion, or blockage, in the coronary arteries of women who were taking estrogen. The protective effect didn't correlate with any of the usual risk factors for the disease except high-density lipoprotein (HDL) cholesterol levels. The level of HDL cholesterol (the kind that's thought to be protective) was significantly higher in the women who took estrogen.

"It appears that estrogen maintains a higher level of HDL cholesterol, although no one knows exactly why," says Harvey Gruchow, M.D., associate professor of medicine at the Medical College of Wisconsin. "And HDL seems to have a protective effect against occlusion."

endometrial cancer in people taking postmenopausal estrogen replacements. But endometrial cancer is very treatable and less risky than a hip fracture, which has a very high mortality rate."

If doctors find severe bone loss has already taken place and estrogen doesn't seem feasible, fluoride in combination with calcium might be used to try to reverse the damage. Generally, however, this treatment is not used as the first line of defense against osteoporosis.

CHAPTER 31
New Hope for Sexual Healing

Now there are effective ways to treat two of women's most distressing sexual problems.

Unlike the more tangible devices available to help male sexual problems, treatments for women are usually more along the lines of counseling or psychosexual therapy. This is mostly due to anatomy. The penis is more mechanically complex, and an erection is very visible. In contrast, the primary female response is vaginal lubrication, which is extremely difficult to measure and study scientifically.

If a woman has anxious feelings about herself, her partner or sexual intercourse in general, the negative outlook may show up in her body's physical response to making love. A lack of vaginal lubrication may make sex uncomfortable or even painful; a lack of vaginal cooperation (vaginismus) may make sex impossible.

Lack of Lubrication

Stress, minor illness, infections, a mental roadblock, a condition such as diabetes, drugs or advancing age and menopause can all hinder the secretion of lubricating fluid in the vagina. Without it, intercourse can be painful, even making tiny tears in the dry vaginal walls.

For temporary dryness, soothing over-the-counter lubricating jellies can help. But a more extensive problem like the hormonal plunge of menopause may call for an estrogen cream.

"After about three weeks of use," says Albert Altchek, M.D., assistant clinical professor of obstetrics, gynecology and reproductive science at Mount Sinai School of Medicine in New York City, "a vaginally inserted estrogen cream can soften, moisten and even thicken the weakened walls of the vagina, as well as reduce any cracks from damaging penile entry. We're even starting to see some evidence that the treatment may help incontinence by improving the urethral walls." (Some women may be at risk for side effects from estrogen, and this cream does get absorbed into the system. A woman's doctor can determine whether she should use the cream.)

Vaginismus

Vaginismus is an involuntary spasm of the muscles surrounding the opening of the vagina and the outer third of the vagina; it can occur as a reaction to imagined, anticipated or real attempts at penetration.

"The fear of being hurt or injured is a major contributing cause," says noted sex and marital therapist Shirley Zussman, Ed.D., codirector of the Association for Male Sexual Dysfunction. "Organic causes that may produce the pain need to be corrected first, but the roots of vaginismus can often be traced in therapy to an inhibiting background concerning sex.

"Having negative sexual attitudes pounded in by parents since childhood, or too rigidly following the dictates of a strict, disapproving religion are two examples of what can inhibit a woman's sexuality and cause this particular dysfunction," Dr. Zussman says. "Or the reason may be intimacy problems: The woman has trouble trusting others, is emotionally guarded and not sexually responsive."

In any case, the impact of vaginismus can be dramatic. Men may develop impotence when every attempt at making love is futile. It's not unusual for therapists to see clients whose marriages have never been consummated because of it. Leading sex researchers William Masters, M.D., and Virginia Johnson point to an unconsummated marriage in 1 out of every 12 clients they see; Dr. Zussman's estimate of the frequency is similar.

Women used to be labeled frigid when they brought this problem to professional attention. Today, the key to treating vaginismus is to help a woman overcome some of her fears and anxieties and learn to relax her vaginal muscle and stretch the vaginal outlet. This is done with physical and psychological approaches.

"Vaginismus is the body reacting to taboos and fears," Dr. Zussman says. "Like the eyes when a finger approaches, it automatically shuts to avoid pain."

A woman can do special exercises to overcome this fear. Therapists have developed a program using plastic, rubber or glass dilators in graduated sizes. A woman begins with the smallest-size dilator and, after a warm bath to relax tissues, gently inserts it to stretch the vagina. This is done several times a day, until the largest dilator can be comfortably inserted. Once she can accept her partner doing this to her, she may soon be tolerant of penile insertion. Fingers can be used instead of the dilators.

The other phase of treatment is psychotherapy. "Vaginismus is, after all, the classic example of a psychosomatic condition—the mind has trouble and unconsciously influences the body to react also," notes Dr. Zussman.

The focus in therapy is to give a woman permission to let go and develop new attitudes about herself and her sexuality. Uncovering her past sexual upbringing is a crucial first step.

Basic anatomy education is probably needed in therapy as well, as it was usually withheld from women with vaginismus. Dr. Zussman recalls one woman who, married for eight years without having intercourse, didn't know where her vagina was.

"Both men and women usually do very well and gain a satisfying sex life after therapy," says Dr. Zussman. "Just talking about the sexual problem is therapeutic; for many, it's the first time they've ever talked about it at all. Everyone feels better once they realize a sex problem is not as scary or embarrassing as they had thought. And after this is accomplished, a normal sex life is close at hand."

CHAPTER 32

Is Cervical Cancer Sexually Transmitted?

New clues to the origin of this disease may help you prevent it.

Why do virgins, nuns and lesbians almost never have abnormal Pap smears? Why are monogamous wives of men who visit prostitutes at high risk for cervical cancer, while women who use barrier contraceptives such as the diaphragm or condom remain at low risk? Researchers are beginning to understand the answers to these baffling questions, and the evidence points to the virus that causes venereal warts (condyloma) as the main culprit.

The Link with Genital Warts

The early precancerous stages of cervical cancer now appear to be a sexually transmitted disease (STD). Several types of sexually transmitted wart viruses have recently been closely linked to the growth of cervical cancer. Presently, more than 30 types of human wart viruses have been isolated, and several of them are associated with warts in the genital area. Most genital warts are caused by viral strains that do not cause cervical cancer. Unfortunately, at present, the average doctor cannot tell if a patient's warts caused by a viral strain are associated with cervical cancer.

When cervical cancer is viewed as a sexually transmitted disease, the low risk experienced by nuns, virgins and lesbians makes sense. Since they do not have intercourse, the wart virus never comes in contact with the cervix. (Lesbians and nuns who have had sex with men in the past may have acquired the infection at that time.) Monogamous women with monogamous partners in groups such as the Mormons, Amish and Seventh-Day Adventists are also at low risk for cervical cancer. Monogamous women whose partners are not monogamous or women who have had multiple sexual relationships significantly increase their risk of cervical cancer, as do women who began sexual relations in their teens, a time when the cervix may be more vulnerable. Since the relaxation of sexual mores in the mid-1960s, genital wart infections have increased sixfold. This increase may result in a dramatic increase in cervical cancer unless women continue to be vigilant about annual Pap smears.

One positive note in the wart/cervical cancer scenario is that women who use a diaphragm or condoms receive considerable protection from the wart virus infection (and other STDs). Numerous studies from family planning clinics have demonstrated the protective effect these barrier methods of contraception have against cervical cancer.

A number of factors may promote the growth of cervical cancer once it's been initiated by the wart virus. Some studies have shown that long-term use of the Pill (four years or more) is associated with more rapid growth of cervical cancers. Counterbalancing this increased risk is the fact that Pill users are more likely to have regular checkups and annual Pap smears, so any cervical abnormality is more likely to be detected early and treated successfully.

Recent studies have also shown that cigarette smokers suffer more cervical cancer. The inhaled toxins in cigarette smoke presumably circulate throughout the body and affect cells that are far distant from the lungs. (Cigarette smokers also have more cancer of the bladder, kidneys, pancreas and other organs.)

Prevention and Early Detection

How can you protect yourself from the wart virus and subsequent cervical cancer? Here are a few suggestions.

Use barrier contraceptives. The condom and diaphragm are associated with lower rates of abnormal Pap smears. If you use another type of contraception such as the Pill, the IUD, the sponge or the rhythm method, consider switching to a barrier contraceptive, especially if you develop abnormal Pap smear results. Shielding the cervix may allow the abnormality to regress.

Have an annual Pap smear. This is important particularly if you are sexually active with men or have been so in the past. Lesbians or celibate women who have had a normal Pap result for two years in a row can generally wait two years between Paps. Consult your clinician about frequency of Pap smears.

Don't ignore an abnormal Pap test. Many precancerous conditions can be eradicated by superficial freezing or laser techniques that don't affect your fertility.

Have genital warts removed. If you or your partner develops genital warts, have a clinician remove them. If a woman develops cervical cancer or its precursors, her male partner(s) should be carefully checked for warts by a health professional. Sometimes these can only be seen on the male by using magnification, so an experienced dermatologist or urologist should be consulted.

Don't smoke. This is particularly important if you have or have had an abnormal Pap smear.

Eat foods rich in folate and vitamins A and C. The American Cancer Society and many researchers say that a diet rich in deep-colored vegetables and fruits may help prevent cervical cancer.

CHAPTER 33

Medical Update: What to Do about Breast Lumps

Now there are effective ways to detect and treat them.

It's difficult to determine how common breast lumps are in women because many lumps are never seen by a doctor. Some cysts are temporary and disappear spontaneously. It's impossible to estimate the number of women seen in a doctor's office for breast lumps. Some estimates indicate up to 25 percent of all visits to a gynecologist are for breast lumps. These are statistics only from lumps that were biopsied and reported by doctors. We really don't know how common the surgery is.

During childbearing years, about two-thirds of all breast lumps are noncancerous (benign). About half of the breast lumps are benign around menopause, and the majority of lumps occurring after menopause are cancerous (malignant).

A lump in the breast can be a single cyst (a tissue sac filled with fluid), a solid mass of tissue, a "lumpiness" throughout the breast (as found with fibrocystic disease) or many degrees in between. A cystic mass may become infected and form an abscess. A lump can be cancerous or noncancerous. A solid tumor may also be surrounded by, or encased in, fluid.

Lumps can be called by many other names, including cyst, mass, tumor, abscess, Ca (abbreviation for carcinoma or cancer), induration, thickening, swelling, enlargement or growth. They affect only the breasts, except when cancer is present or there is an abscess or infection, when lymph glands under the arm may be swollen. If your cyst is cancerous, the cancer may spread elsewhere in the body. It usually begins to spread to lymph glands under the arm and often spreads to the opposite breast. Cancer may also spread to the bones, liver, lungs or brain. It usually spreads to organs where there is a rich blood supply to support its rapid growth.

Self-Detection

We know that 90 percent of all breast lumps are discovered by women themselves, not by their doctors. This places most of the responsibility on you to examine yourself thoroughly and often. Here are some suggestions to help you become proficient at examining your own breasts for lumps.

When? Examine your breasts once a month, preferably right after your menstrual period, when fullness and tenderness are no longer present.

Where? Do it in the tub or shower, because the "wet" feel appears to be more accurate. Fingers slide more easily over wet skin. Or do it lying down.

How? Use the palm of your hand and the flat part of your fingers as you examine each part of each breast with a circular, almost "massaging" motion.

Examine all of the breast. Divide each breast into four quadrants—upper, lower, left and right. Examine each quadrant of each breast. Keep in mind that the upper-outer quadrant (toward your armpit) is most likely to contain cancerous lumps.

Normally you have some small lymph nodes under your arms. If the glands are enlarged enough to be easily outlined, check with your doctor. There is a projection of breast tissue that extends under your armpit, which means any lump could be breast tissue rather than an enlarged lymph gland. Infection also causes enlarged lymph nodes in your armpit, including infection anywhere within your arm or breast.

Do a mirror inspection. Stand or sit in front of a mirror and inspect your breasts. Sometimes cancer causes an obvious bulge. Certain cancers retract tissue and may cause dimpling of the breast.

Look for any lesion that pulls, pushes or distorts the nipple in any way. Any chronically sore nipple that won't heal should be examined by your doctor for Paget's disease (cancer of the nipple and surrounding area).

It's common for one breast to be larger than the other. But if your breasts have appeared to be equal in size in the past and now show a discrepancy, check for the presence of a lump in the larger breast.

Examine your breasts when you're standing or sitting. When standing, you may discover something in your breasts that you didn't find when you checked them lying down.

Check for discharge. There should be no discharge from your nipple, especially a bloody or foul-smelling one. You should not be able to express any discharge from your nipple.

Practice examining your breasts. You should become familiar with the contour, texture and density of your breasts. If you think you feel a lump in one breast, check to see if there is a similar mass in the opposite breast. It's uncommon to have a solitary lump in each breast, especially in the same location.

Sleep on your stomach occasionally. Many women discover a lump in their breast while sleeping face-down. They say they feel as if they are lying on a marble or some other object. If you don't sleep on your stomach regularly, do it occasionally to see if you feel any unusual lumps.

All lumps are important and must be diagnosed as to type and cause. If you feel a lump in your breast, don't try to second-guess it. Have it examined immediately by your doctor. The only way to reduce the high number of breast cancers that spread by the time they are detected is to discover them earlier!

If you discover a lump just before or during your menstrual period, watch to see if it disappears as your period subsides. If it persists, even beyond one menstrual period, have it examined by your doctor.

If you discover a round, regular breast mass, it may be a cyst. Your doctor may decide to try to withdraw fluid from it with a syringe. If he withdraws fluid and the mass completely disappears, it was a cyst, and there is no cause for concern. Aspirated (withdrawn) fluid is sent to a lab to be examined for any suspicious cells.

If your doctor can't aspirate any fluid or if there is still a mass, even though it's smaller after he has aspirated all the fluid possible, the remaining lump must be biopsied to rule out cancer. Don't ignore any breast lump!

A Roll Call of Benign Lumps

There are several different types of benign breast lumps that you should know about.

Fibroadenoma. This is a common, benign breast lump that usually appears in young women and occasionally in adolescents. It's a painless, freely movable, firm tumor that may become large. These masses almost always appear in groups, and often they are found in both breasts.

Perhaps the greatest problem that a fibroadenoma causes is your worry that it might be malignant. Because it occurs most often in younger women and because cancer is rarely found in women under age 25, the worry is usually unwarranted. Under the age of 25, fibroadenomas can be safely observed and do not demand immediate biopsy.

Fibrocystic disease. This term means that your breast contains many cysts, which can keep you constantly worried about whether any of these "lumps" might be cancerous. In fact, 35 to 50 percent of all women have fibrocystic disease at some time during their lives.

It is usually found in both breasts and is often in multiples: there may be countless cysts. Sometimes the condition produces a feeling of "lumpiness" in the breasts.

Typically, fibrocystic disease produces a dull, heavy pain. It often causes a feeling of fullness and tenderness that increases each month just before the onset of your menstrual period and becomes more tolerable after your period. Cysts become larger and more tender, then decrease in size and tenderness.

These cysts are often easy to locate and outline with your fingers. They are tender to the touch. Deeper clusters of cysts are more worrisome and are more likely to be biopsied, often repeatedly. Usually larger breast cysts can be aspirated with a syringe and needle, but deeper cysts lead to scarred breasts from repeated biopsies.

In some cases, the problem becomes so worrisome that all breast tissue is removed, leaving the skin intact. An artificial breast, made of a silicone-gel envelope, is inserted in its place.

Certain types of fibrocystic disease have no relationship to breast cancer; others are suspect. It requires all your doctor's skill and sometimes several diagnostic methods to be certain.

Intraductal papilloma. This is another small, benign tumor. It is found in a milk duct and can produce a clear, milky or bloody discharge from your nipple. Usually, no tumor mass is found.

Only rarely are these tumor masses cancerous, but they are of concern to you. Discharge from your breast should be examined microscopically for cancer cells. A mammogram should also be done.

If your breast discharge persists, the papilloma must be removed because of its nuisance factor. But these tumors are almost always benign.

Ductal ectasia. This term means blocked, stretched, swollen or dilated breast ducts. Ductal ectasia is characterized by a sticky, multicolored discharge from your nipple that causes burning and itching around the nipple and areola.

Along with a drawing, dull pain, you can often feel tender, tubular swellings under the areola. If these swellings increase in size, they may be confused with cancer, although they are definitely benign.

In some cases, all the breast tissue is removed, leaving the skin intact. A silicone-gel envelope is inserted in its place.

About Breast Surgery

Needle aspiration of cysts can be done in a doctor's office, often with only a small amount of local anesthetic. If the mass disappears after withdrawal of the fluid, your problem is solved.

If a mass is still present, it may have to be biopsied. But the doctor first probes with the needle to make certain it isn't another cyst. If the fluid is blood-tinged, it is more suspicious because it may also contain cancer cells from a cancer in the cyst.

In needle biopsy of a solid tumor, a special large biopsy needle is inserted into your breast lump to extract tissue for examination and diagnosis in the lab.

In a lumpectomy (a kind of biopsy), an attempt is made to remove the entire lump. Unless the tumor is too far removed from your nipple, a semicircular incision is made in the outer edge of the areola. The mass is cut free, and the incision is closed. The incision is compressed with pressure bandages for several hours after surgery. The advantage of an incision that follows the border of the areola is that your scar is scarcely visible.

There's also a biopsy in which only part of a lump is removed. This type of biopsy is done when it seems certain your tumor is malignant or if for some other reason it cannot be removed completely in the office or in outpatient surgery.

The risk of a biopsy or complete removal of breast lumps is very low. A radical mastectomy—removal of the breast with wide dissection that includes underlying muscles and overlying skin, removal of lymph nodes under the arm and fatty tissue—is massive and carries significant risks of complications in up to 50 percent of all cases.

This operation is rapidly being replaced by simple lumpectomy and postoperative radiation. Results with a radical operation have always been severe, hazardous, disabling and disfiguring. By contrast, a lumpectomy is relatively simple and safe and, in many instances, may be as effective for cure as the radical approach, when followed by radiation.

Most women would rather have several biopsies that showed only a benign mass than miss the one cancerous mass that could be successfully treated if biopsied early. Your cure rate soars from 46 percent to over 80 percent if cancer of the breast is discovered early, *before* it has time to spread.

There are no disadvantages to having a biopsy of your breast. Regardless of the number of benign biopsies, it's worth it to avoid the tragedy of cancer in a breast lump that is observed instead of biopsied. The only possible exception is when you have fibrocystic disease with multiple cysts in each breast. Even these lumps must be aspirated to remove the fluid and make certain no residual mass is present.

On rare occasions, if cysts become too numerous, too deep in your breast to examine or too worrisome, it may become necessary to remove all of your breast tissue, leaving the skin intact. The diseased breast tissue can be replaced with a silicone-gel implant. This dispels the worry, avoids frequent biopsies and does not disfigure the contour of your breast. This is called prophylactic subcutaneous mastectomy. However, this procedure performed on a fibrocystic breast simply to remove the threat of cancer is condemned as unwarranted and unnecessary surgery. If your doctor suggests this operation, obtain a second opinion from a breast center or cancer specialist.

If a simple biopsy or breast aspiration is anticipated, your family physician, obstetrician or general surgeon may perform the operation. The same might apply to a simple lumpectomy.

If more radical treatment is needed, a general surgeon usually performs the surgery. If all the breast tissue is to be removed because of chronic fibrocystic disease and a prosthesis inserted, a plastic surgeon is the person most qualified to do this. As stated previously, you should get a second opinion before having such an operation.

Risking Cancer

The true risk lies not in the surgery but in what is found at surgery. Whether your lesion is benign or malignant, immediate healing and recovery seem uneventful. If your lump is malignant, further treatment depends on the type of cancer, whether it can be destroyed by x-ray, whether it has spread to other parts of the body and, if so, how extensively.

The risk lies in the possibility and extent of malignancy. Figures vary depending on the population, but 1 in 11 women in the United States develops breast cancer in her lifetime. The majority of tumors are discovered by women themselves. Doctors uncover only 10 percent of all breast cancers. Of all the major cancers in women (except for lung cancer), only breast cancer has had no decrease in mortality in the past 50 years.

When we study these statistics, we quickly realize our greatest hope lies in diagnosing breast cancer earlier. At present, more than 50 percent of breast cancers have spread beyond local limits by the time they are discovered. This points up the importance and urgency of finding ways to diagnose breast cancer earlier.

Certain women are more likely than others to develop breast cancer. If you have had no children, you're more likely to have breast cancer. The same applies if you have your first child after age 27. If you have your first child after age 34, you are four times more prone to have breast cancer.

Breastfeeding was thought to protect women against breast cancer. Actually, it gives protection only if you nurse your baby for more than 36 months.

Heredity is a factor in breast cancer. Breast cancer in your mother or sister increases your relative risk three times. This risk increases to five times if both your mother and your grandmother had breast cancer.

Obesity is thought to increase the risk of breast cancer. When combined with high blood pressure and diabetes, obesity increases the risk three times.

In most studies conducted since 1970, it has been concluded that there is no relationship between estrogen and breast cancer, whether the hormone is taken before, during or after menopause, and whether it is given alone or in combination with other drugs, such as birth control pills. There is some evidence that oral contraceptives may even have a slight protective benefit in reducing the risk of breast cancer. One study indicates that if oral contraceptives are used for more than four years, they may reduce your risk of breast cancer by as much as 50 percent.

If you have had cancer in one breast, you are five times as likely to develop cancer in your other breast. Check yourself frequently and have regular exams by your physician, along with mammography.

If you have significant fibrocystic disease of the breast, you are two to four times more likely to develop cancer of the breast, although not in the cysts. Check your breasts regularly and have regular exams.

High-Tech Detection of Breast Lumps

There are methods that detect cancer before a lump can be felt. These procedures are called screening for breast cancer. By the time a cancer is large enough to be discovered by a woman, enough of the cancer may have spread so that only about 50 percent of the women can have hope of a five-year cure. We must discover breast cancer *before* you can feel it if we hope to improve the cure rates.

There are more than a dozen different methods of examining breasts other than by "feeling," or palpation, during a physical exam. Every method cannot, and should not, be used on every woman. Here are some of them.

Heat-sensing techniques. The human body gives off electromagnetic waves within the infrared spectrum. These waves are influenced by the temperature of your tissues. Irritated, infected tissues give off more heat, and so does tissue that contains cancer. Radiation of heat can be measured and recorded like we record an x-ray image.

There are various methods, but we'll call all of them thermography.

The trouble with thermography in detecting early cancers is that it yields too many false positives and false negatives. Hopefully, use of the computer may make this method more accurate. At present, we can't rely on thermography when used alone. But one study showed that the accuracy of x-ray mammography is increased when combined with thermography on the same patient at the same time.

Ultrasound mammography. Ultrasound is sound waves "echoed off" tissue of your breast; these sound waves can be recorded. Although there seems to be little risk with ultrasonography, its usefulness in screening for breast cancer is minimal at this time. It can help detect benign cysts in your breast that can be drained to rule out breast cancer, but it has very limited use.

Light transmission. The medical term is diaphanography, but it means shining a very intense, cool light through your breast and noting the shadow it casts. This light can be recorded on film. Light transmission is a helpful tool, but it is not very accurate when compared with x-ray mammography.

Nuclear magnetic resonance (NMR). NMR is also called nuclear magnetic imaging (NMI). Explained simply, an entire room is converted into a huge magnet. You are placed in the room, and radio waves are directed toward the magnetic field. The nuclei of your tissues align themselves temporarily, according to the magnetic field, and form an image that can be recorded. Breast tumors show up well. This is proving to be an effective way to distinguish harmless lumps from those that must be removed.

Equipment for this type of testing costs from half a million dollars to several million dollars. But this method, which in time will become less expensive, simpler and more available, promises to be an extremely sensitive method for early detection of breast cancer.

X-ray mammography. We often combine methods and variations in methods, but at present, x-ray mammography is our best screening tool. In fact, one large study showed the fatality rate from breast cancer was reduced by as much as 33 percent by mammographic screening. Techniques have improved since then, and mortality rates could be reduced even more using these improvements.

X-ray mammography offers excellent help in early diagnosis, but its use is individualized. Mammography involves radiation, so it should not be used routinely in young women. It is now recommended annually for asymptomatic women over 50 years of age, with a baseline mammogram done between the ages of 35 and 40. Also, women between the ages of 40 and 50 should have an exam every two years; some doctors and researchers recommend it be done every year.

Recommendations are different for younger women with a family history of breast cancer or other high risk factors, as previously discussed. Talk about your concerns with your doctor.

All suspicious lesions that show up on mammograms should be biopsied. Some may be as small as a cantaloupe seed. Other mammograms may show only calcification. Suspicious lesions that persist on mammograms must be biopsied, even though they are probably benign.

This practice may lead to more biopsies of benign lesions, but malignant lesions will be discovered earlier. Your life could be saved by these precautions.

PART VIII: BETTER WAYS TO BEAT EVERYDAY HEALTH PROBLEMS

CHAPTER 34

The Nine Causes of Fatigue and How to Overcome Them

If it feels like you've about given up the ghost, here's how you can revive your sagging spirit, and your body along with it.

"Tell the kids to answer their own phone calls, or hire temporary office help. Get somebody else to change the toilet-paper roll and pick up the dirty socks. Let the dog walk himself."

Sound familiar? If you're barking at the dog and the bags under your eyes are so big they qualify as carry-on luggage, maybe you're just running on empty. We all know the feeling, that weary-down-to-your-bones sensation of fatigue. When you're feeling that low, it's hard to be high on life, let alone pick up socks. But it doesn't have to be that way. You can banish fatigue and reinvigorate that energetic old you.

Fatigue can be an early clue that your emotions are out of kilter. It can also be a signal of a physical illness.

We've assembled a list of nine of the most common causes of fatigue. If you feel run-down, here's the low-down.

1. Not enough sleep. It seems so obvious, but if you haven't slept well the night before, you're very likely going to feel tired the day after.

Half of all Americans have trouble dozing off at some time in their lives, and an astonishing 35 million of us have chronic insomnia. Scientists believe sleep disturbance is a common response to change in our lives, from trouble at the office to serious illness. For most of us, normal sleep patterns return after the daytime problem that is the source of worry goes away or gets better.

If occasional sleeplessness troubles you, follow these simple suggestions from Patricia Prinz, Ph.D., associate professor of psychiatry and behavioral sciences at the University of Washington School of Medicine.

- Try not to drink coffee, cola or other caffeine drinks after 6:00 or 7:00 P.M.
- Go to bed at the same time every night.
- Get regular, moderate exercise.
- Skip alcohol after dinner. Booze interferes with sound sleep.

2. Poor nutrition. They don't call them "crash" diets for nothing. Diet or not, you have to eat if you don't want to wind up nose-down on the pavement. Simply put, crash or fad diets can leave you feeling fatigued.

Because they offer so little in the way of balanced nutrition, crash diets can turn your muscle mass into mush. The destruction becomes so pronounced, after a short time, that the muscle tissue can no longer efficiently process calcium, according to studies done at the University of Toronto. If you're on that kind of diet, your body will not be able to function properly. It will slow down and conserve energy by making you slow down.

To get a good start on a diet that will leave you feeling fresh and exhilarated, bear in mind these basic rules.

- Eat a variety of foods. Avoid diet plans that force you to live on one specific kind of food, like grapefruit. We need a wide variety of nutrients from all kinds of food. No one food supplies you with all the nutrients your body needs to maintain health.
- Women in general shouldn't eat fewer than 1,200 calories a day; men, not less than 1,500 calories. According to diet and nutrition experts at Stanford University, you can't get all the nutrients you need if you eat less than those amounts. Diets in the super-low 800-calorie range may pose a particular threat to health, which can result in a breakdown in heart muscle.
- If you cut 250 calories a day from your diet, you should lose about a half a pound a week.
- Don't eat big meals late at night. You probably won't be able to burn off the calories as quickly by bedtime as you would earlier in the day.
- Don't skip meals. If you do, you'll only be hungrier later. When you do sit down to eat, you probably will eat more than you should.

3. Lack of exercise. If your body isn't exercised regularly, it probably doesn't use oxygen very efficiently. Your muscles need that oxygen, or they won't work as long or as hard as they can. The result of all this sitting around: When you need muscle power, you don't get it, and you tire quickly.

What's more, even as your muscles sag, so does your self-image. Your emotional state can become a mirror image of your physical condition, adding to your fatigue.

That's why exercise benefits you in two ways. First, it improves your physical condition, enabling your body to more efficiently deliver oxygen to your muscles, increasing your endurance. Second, exercise stimulates an overall feeling of well-being.

Studies show that as you exercise, your body becomes better able to handle the everyday emotional and physical stresses of life, says Ralph Wharton, M.D., clinical professor of psychiatry at Columbia University. "The question is, what does exercise do in a neurochemical sense? We don't know exactly," he says. "But we do know that, whatever exercise does for the brain, it also seems to do for the ego. When people exercise, they see themselves running or swimming. They feel a certain mastery of the environment."

4. Drug reactions. You get plenty of sleep, you jog around the park, but you still feel exhausted, like you just can't get started. Maybe your fatigue is coming from outside your body.

A number of drugs—including antihistamines, pain relievers, diuretics, antihypertensives, antibiotics, oral contraceptives and anticonvulsants—can sometimes cause fatigue as a side effect.

If you are taking a drug and you think it makes you feel drowsy, the first thing to do is to call the pharmacist who sold you the product, says William N. Tindall, Ph.D., director of professional affairs for the National Association of Retail Druggists.

"The pharmacist will have your complete drug history and will be able to tell whether the drug you are taking is causing your drowsiness, or whether two drugs in combination are having that effect. Then the pharmacist will call the doctor and, together, they'll decide the best thing to do," he says.

What they might do, says Dr. Tindall, is substitute another drug. "With all the drugs on the market, they can usually find something that isn't as hard on the patient."

Whatever you do, don't stop taking a prescription drug without consulting your physician first.

5. Stress. It takes a lot of energy to deal with the pressures of everyday life. After expending all that energy, you may be left with a gnawing, overwhelming sense of fatigue.

Not all the stresses of life leave us feeling emotionally drained. "It takes a certain kind of stress, in which you have no choices, no options, no alternatives," says Harvey L. Alpern, M.D., a board-certified cardiologist in Los Angeles. "The classic example is the woman who finds herself in a dead-end job. She has a tough boss that she can't talk back to. She has to do the same repetitive thing day after day. She has no sense of control. She may have a family who needs her, so she has even more work to do when she gets home. She is trapped. This woman may suffer fatigue."

If you're stuck in that kind of situation, maybe it seems like there's nothing you can do. But according to Dr. Alpern, the symptoms of fatigue associated with stress can often be alleviated by doing the following things.

- Ask your doctor or consult a stress therapist about relaxation techniques. They may only take 10 or 15 minutes to learn.
- Once you know the techniques, use them to take a couple of 10- or 15-minute "vacations" from your work around the home or office every day. "Doing these exercises and paying attention to your feelings can break that all-day feeling of tension," says Dr. Alpern.

6. Anemia. Take the iron out of a bridge, and it will collapse. Run low on iron in your blood, and maybe you'll collapse. Iron deficiency can lead to anemia, which in turn can lead to fatigue.

Even if your diet is iron-rich, you might have trouble holding onto it. In women, heavy menstrual flow may deplete the body's stores of iron, resulting in frequent fatigue, says James D. Cook, M.D., head of the Division of Hematology at the University of Kansas Medical Center. Men, on the other hand, may suffer iron deficiency due to gastrointestinal bleeding. Such bleeding might be virtually unnoticeable yet sufficient to cause anemia.

Pregnant women and children going through rapid growth periods often need more iron than the rest of us. If this need is not met, they, too, may have iron-deficiency anemia and that washed-out feeling.

The U.S. Recommended Daily Allowance (USRDA) of iron for adults and children over four years of age is 18 milligrams. Among the best food sources of iron are beef liver, dark meat turkey, lean ground beef, lima beans, sunflower seeds, prunes, broccoli and spinach. If you're supplementing, stick to the USRDA unless your doctor tells you otherwise. Iron in large amounts can be harmful.

7. Diabetes. Chronic weariness, along with thirst and general weakness, can signify the onset of diabetes. Nonstop fatigue might also be the first sign of hepatitis, a thyroid disorder, mononucleosis, tuberculosis or infection.

"More often than not, emotional factors of stress or depression are the cause of fatigue," says Dr. Alpern. But if you do feel tired all the time, even right after you get up in the morning, call your doctor for a checkup.

8. Heart disease. One of the first warning signs of heart disease—and occasionally, the only signal—may be fatigue.

"The word *fatigue,* to a cardiologist, is very important," says Dr. Alpern. "Fatigue is one of the things we look for in the person in his fifties or sixties as a possible warning sign of an impending heart attack. Fatigue may be associated with a change in the heart, so it is a good reason to get in for a checkup, particularly in the age group we're talking about."

What to do about fatigue, in this situation, may not be as simple. A heart problem, obviously, calls for immediate medical intervention. If you feel tired all the time, or if you have any other symptoms of heart attack, such as squeezing chest pain below the breastbone, general weakness or nausea, seek medical help without delay.

9. Depression. Your only son is about to marry an intelligent, beautiful young woman. She's the kind of person you would have picked yourself for someone as special as your boy. There's every reason for joy in your life, but that's not how you feel. You're very sad and very tired. And, suddenly, this wedding is becoming a problem.

"Fatigue often is a warning signal of a failure to master a problem," says Dr. Wharton. "Sometimes there is anticipation of a conflict, and other times the conflict is ongoing."

Another reason why a depressed person might feel exhausted is lack of sleep. "Many depressed people may have serious trouble sleeping," says Dr. Wharton, "or they'll have recurring nightmares. The sleep disturbance is part of the depressive cycle. They'll wake up feeling tired.

In fact, they've been sleeping, but they've been having very troublesome dreams, which can be as exhausting as if they were struggling during the day, digging a ditch. They're digging a deeper and deeper hole and never getting out of it."

But you can start getting out of this hole if you begin to understand why you feel depressed. "It's often possible to see what you can do to prevent trouble in the future, to prevent this fatigue reaction that makes everything an effort," says Dr. Wharton.

But there's more to getting better than recognizing what makes you depressed. Once you know the underlying cause of your emotional downturn, you then have to change the way you react to the situation. For either option, you might need the emotional help of a trained mental health practitioner.

"Sometimes, getting better means taking a look at how you have dealt with crises in the past and learning ways to deal with the new crisis," says Dr. Wharton. "Other times, it requires an exploration of one's whole past. But the good news is that fatigue of this sort is usually treatable."

Whatever the cause of your fatigue, it's important to obtain an expert diagnosis. Your weariness could be the result of simple muscle fatigue, stress, lack of exercise or, says Dr. Alpern, "just about any disease the body could get, from a cold to the worst." Fortunately, most fatigue is not serious. But if you have chronic unexplained fatigue, ask your doctor for help.

CHAPTER 35
25 Ways to Whip Your Allergies

Here is practical, up-to-the-minute advice to help you snuff the sniffles and nix the itch.

Whoever said life isn't fair must have been thinking about allergies.

Some of us can plow through thickets of poison ivy and emerge without an itch. If others so much as brush up against a few spindly sprigs of the stuff, they're digging holes through their panty hose for weeks. For the majority of people, happiness is a warm puppy, yet dog fur brings thousands to heel. Why?

The reason is a difference in the sensitivity of the immune system. Burdened with an overprotective immune system, a person with allergies is forever on guard against everyday things that don't bother the rest of us. It might be a slice of fresh garden tomato or a patch of clover, a glass of milk or an affectionate kitten.

In most instances, allergies are more annoying than debilitating. Coping often involves avoiding foods to which you might be sensitive or taking an antihistamine to dry up the occasional runny nose and soothe the itchy eyes of hay fever.

No matter what type of allergy you have, there's a good chance you can find relief. Here are 25 of the best tips, based on the latest research and interviews with allergy experts.

1. Avoid foods that trigger migraines. Up to one-third of all migraines may be caused by food allergies, according to Lyndon E. Mansfield, M.D., clinical associate professor at Texas Tech University Health Sciences Center.

The most common food trigger of migraines is wheat, followed by corn, peanuts and soybeans, with milk causing the most headaches in children.

But when these foods are avoided, says Dr. Mansfield, some people (but not all) may have fewer headaches, less painful migraines or no headaches at all.

If your headaches have been diagnosed as migraines, consult an allergist for tests to discover if you have food allergies.

2. Don't pierce young ears. There's been an upsurge in allergic reactions to the metal nickel, particularly among girls under 15 who have had their ears pierced. In fact, nickel allergy is the most common contact allergy among women. The metal pins worn for the first three to six weeks after piercing contain minute quantities of nickel, which makes the body vulnerable to rashes later when the metal comes in contact with skin. Reactions are common with jewelry, metal buttons, wristwatches, brassieres and and eyeglass frames.

Studies also show that girls with more than one hole in the ear, as in the current "pincushion" look, have twice as many allergies. Researchers advise against ear piercing in children.

3. Chew or sip more slowly. Sulfites are chemicals used to treat foods to make them look fresh. The U.S. Food and Drug Administration (FDA) has banned the use of these chemicals in supermarket produce or restaurant salad bars because they have induced fatal allergic reactions in people with asthma.

But we aren't rid of sulfites altogether. The FDA ban does not apply to prepared foods, such as potato products, frozen and canned vegetables, wine, beer, seafood, dried fruit, dry-mix salad dressings and soups.

Asthmatics and others who could be allergic to sulfites might be able to control an allergic reaction simply by eating or drinking more slowly. Up to 90 percent of sulfite reactions result from the release of sulfur dioxide gas from food, caused by chewing and sipping, according to Ronald Simon, M.D., a member of the FDA's advisory group on food additives. The allergic reaction is the result of inhaling sulfur dioxide. Many asthmatics have learned to drink and eat more slowly and to watch for the warning signs of a reaction—itching, warmth, flushing, chest congestion, abdominal discomfort, coughing and wheezing.

4. Tell your dentist about your allergies. Nickel and sulfite allergies also surface in the dentist's office. Fillings, dentures, caps, braces and crowns may contain nickel. Local anesthetics also may be preserved with a sulfite chemical. If you're allergic to either substance, the dentist ought to be told before he goes to work in your mouth.

5. Avoid eyeglass rash. Spray a polyurethane coating on eyeglass frames occasionally to avoid the itchy facial rash caused by the interaction of sweat with eyeglass materials.

6. Keep Kitty off the bed. Cat got your nose? Could be she's been sleeping in your bed. Kitty's attachment to your bedcovers increases the amount of allergy-producing substances in your sleeping quarters a thousandfold. You don't have to hide your felines, though—just keep them out of your bedroom. The same rule applies to Rover.

Additionally, if you can get your pets used to spending more time outdoors, you'll greatly reduce the number of animal allergens—the microscopic particles that touch off your allergic reactions—in your house. Outdoors is also a good place to brush and pet your cat or dog.

7. Switch sunscreens. If sunscreen on your shoulder makes you rashy, you might be allergic to para-aminobenzoic acid (PABA).

PABA is present not only in many commercial sunscreens but in cosmetics as well. So it doesn't have to be summer for you to be affected.

To find out whether PABA turns your skin itchy and red, try a patch test first. Dab some PABA-containing lotion on a section of skin not normally exposed to the sun. Apply it twice a day for three days. If your skin doesn't break out, repeat the test on an exposed patch of flesh—the back of your hand is a good place. If you still don't react, you can probably use PABA without problems.

If you *do* react, try one of the many alternative sunscreens, such as benzophenone, sulsibenzone, oxybenzone, cinnamate compounds or the PABA derivative octyldimethyl PABA.

8. Squelch that smoke. Cigarette smoke is bad enough, but for asthmatics, it could cause serious breathing difficulties. Secondhand cigarette smoke greatly increases the likelihood of an asthma attack for up to four hours, according to Australian researchers. Smoke evidently makes the asthmatic more sensitive to other allergens, such as dust, cold air or exercise, they add.

Just leaving the smoke-filled room may not be enough. By the time you make your exit, it could be too late. To avoid the complications caused by smoke, you have to bypass the smoke altogether.

9. For an allergy-free baby, watch your diet. Some babies are born with allergies to foods their mother ate to excess during pregnancy. Oddly enough, some pregnant women crave foods to which they're allergic. If they don't get the food, they develop uncomfortable physical symptoms, like sweating and chills. Should you crave these foods during pregnancy, it might not be possible to avoid them altogether without some discomfort. But try to limit your intake and eat the desired food along with other foods, advises Vincent A. Marinkovich, M.D., a Stanford University pediatric allergist. Don't overdo any one food.

If you've already given birth to one child with a food allergy, he adds, avoid that food during the next pregnancy. Your next baby should be relatively free of food allergies.

10. Put the squeeze on your asthma inhaler. Asthmatics often use metered-dose inhalers to shoot a fine mist of medication into their bronchial tubes. But some people with arthritis or those who have small hands have trouble pushing the button atop the aerosol bottle. Others just have trouble coordinating the effort of pushing down on the top of the bottle and inhaling at the same time.

Glaxo has developed a plastic squeeze trigger called VentEase, which slips over the inhaler to make it easier to use. To get one free, ask your doctor or pharmacist, or call Glaxo's medical department at (800) 334-0089.

11. Sniff for the hidden scent. Cosmetic and grooming aid manufacturers sell a lot of products marked "unscented." But the fragrance may actually be masked with a chemical, ethylene brassalate. If you're allergic to fragrances, beware. Doctors believe you can react to this neutral scent just as easily as you might to any other fragrance. Read the label, and avoid ethylene brassalate.

12. Close your air conditioner vent. An air conditioner can do a lot of good for a person allergic to pollen or fungus spores. But if you keep the vent control in the open position, you're sucking outside air—and pollen—indoors. Pollen is extremely small, so your air conditioner filter probably can't screen it all out. Also, research shows that there is a brief "burst" of mold contamination when the air conditioner is turned on because of mold inside the machine. So turn on the air conditioner and leave the room for half an hour. This will give the molds in the room time to dissipate, resulting in cleaner, more breathable air.

Other people are very sensitive to cold air. So if you have your air conditioner temperature control set to "Arctic" and ice floes are forming in your living room, turn the temperature up to around 70°F.

Automobile air conditioners are subject to the same hazards, so keep the vent closed and run the air conditioner with the car windows open for a few minutes before you get in. And keep the temperature temperate.

13. Allergic to ragweed? Be alert for melon allergy, too. Some people who are allergic to ragweed also develop itching or swelling of the lips, tongue or throat after eating watermelon, cantaloupe, honeydew, zucchini or cucumber. According to the Allergy Research Laboratory Division of Detroit's Henry Ford Hospital, these fruits and vegetables have allergy-producing proteins almost identical to those found in ragweed.

14. Avoid fur-bearin' varmints. If you're allergic to dogs and cats, it's likely you'll also react where the deer and the antelope play. If you're a hunter, that means getting someone else to handle animal carcasses. If you're a "hunter's widow," don't handle your husband's hunting clothes.

15. Go easy on shellfish if you're allergic to shrimp. Chances are pretty good you're also allergic to crayfish, lobster, clams, oysters and crab, according to physicians from the clinical immunology section at Tulane University Medical Center. Common reactions include hives, nausea and shortness of breath.

16. Declare war on dust bunnies. Many people are allergic to substances found within their own homes, particularly dust. But you can keep dust down by doing any one of the following things.

- Have a contractor clean out your heating system. All it takes is a couple of carbon dioxide fire extinguishers and a little time.
- If you're redoing an allergy sufferer's room, forget rugs. Instead, use linoleum—in solid sheets, not blocks. Mold hangs out in the cracks between linoleum blocks.
- If you're wallpapering, purchase mold-free wallpaper paste. If you're painting, have mold preventive added to the paint. It'll cost about $1.50 extra per gallon.
- Finally, when you plaster, look for the one-coat variety that doesn't need sanding.

17. Try this new test for children's food allergies. It's called a MAST test, and it's a great improvement over the uncomfortable standard method of testing for allergies, which involves placing tiny food samples under the child's skin and waiting for a reaction.

For the MAST test, all the doctor needs is a small blood sample, according to Dr. Marinkovich. The MAST test uses a small chamber divided into sections; each section contains a thread coated with a specific allergen. After blood is placed in the chamber, the doctor examines the threads to determine whether antibodies in the blood are reacting to the allergens.

The MAST procedure can detect allergic reactions to 35 different foods. The test is particularly accurate in pinning down children's food allergies. In adults, it is less accurate, because their circulating antibodies are different.

18. Stick to white glue. Many of the new "super" adhesives do dry more quickly and hold better, but some people who use them develop contact dermatitis. A few also develop other allergic reactions, such as asthma.

19. Be satisfied with not-so-soft sheets. Some of the laundry-softener strips cause allergic reactions. For most of us, that may not be a problem, but if you develop a chronic runny nose, coughing and wheezing, asthma or skin rash, fabric softener sheets might be the cause. One manufacturer has investigated 300 such complaints.

20. Consider using an air cleaner. Newer models are very effective at removing dust, pollen, cigarette smoke and mold from the household environment. Cheap models are considerably less effective, according to Harold S. Nelson, M.D., chairman of the American Academy of Allergy and Immunology's Committee on Environmental Controls.

Since an air cleaner can be expensive, Dr. Nelson recommends leasing one first to see if it does the job. Take time to decide if it moves enough air, and try it out in your bedroom for a couple of nights to find out how much noise it makes. When you use a filter, put it in the middle of the room, where it can do the most good.

21. Check out your contact lens solution. If you wear contacts and get itchy, teary or swollen eyes, it could be an allergic reaction to thimersol, a mercury preservative used in contact lens solutions. Another common ingredient, the enzyme papain, can also cause allergic reactions. Switch to a solution that contains neither.

22. Wear an invisible shield against poison oak and poison ivy. A new product, Ivy Block, appears to prevent the sap from these plants from irritating the skin. The spray may not be available over the counter yet, but it is being offered through dermatologists and allergists. Ask about it.

If you don't have such a product and you find yourself exposed to either poison plant, here's what to do, according to William Epstein, M.D., professor of dermatology at the University of California at San Francisco. Wash the affected area immediately with rubbing alcohol, then with water. Wash everything you might have touched with water. And don't use a washrag, since this will also pick up and spread the poison.

23. Observe garden precautions. Yes, you can garden, if you follow a few precautions.

Do your gardening in the evening because most weeds unleash their pollen in the morning. Also, water the soil regularly to keep the dust and mold down, and wear gardening gloves if you have sensitive skin.

24. Be prepared for insect stings. It's hard to believe a tiny insect can do so much damage, but an allergic reaction can lead to anaphylactic shock, which is life-threatening.

If you are sensitive to insect stings, immunotherapy can help. This involves being injected every few weeks with gradually increasing quantities of diluted venom. And you shouldn't stop getting your shots in the winter, says Martin D. Valentine, M.D., professor of medicine at Johns Hopkins University School of Medicine. If you stop during the winter, you'll lose the protection you've built up.

25. Learn to protect yourself against stings. Wear sandals instead of going barefoot. Most stings happen when people tiptoe barefoot through the tulips.

Also, check woodpiles for nests before you start stacking more logs on top. In warmer weather, the same goes for picnic tables.

Finally, shake that beverage can before putting it to your lips. If you hear buzzing inside, either your soda has a short or there's something alive in there. Either way, put it down and bug out.

CHAPTER 36

Four First Aid Moves That Could Save Your Life

There have been a few new twists in emergency care since the time-honored tourniquet.

If you learned first aid back when you were a Scout, you probably know there's more to emergency care than pickling your patient with rye whiskey and wedging a bullet between his teeth.

Like millions of other first aiders, you were taught to cope calmly and rationally with bumps, bruises, cuts and an occasional nosebleed. The skills you learned were taught in easy A-B-C steps, and nothing changed from year to year. Or so you might have thought.

As first aiders went about their business, splinting broken bones and tweezing splinters, medical experts began to wonder about the long-term results of all that well-intentioned care. After years of research, they found that a few of the old skills don't work. They also discovered new skills that are much more effective.

With these new techniques and a few changes in the old skills, they decided, the Good Samaritan could become even better. Here are four of the latest changes in first aid.

Cough for Consciousness

First came cardiopulmonary resuscitation, or CPR, the life-saving marriage of external chest massage and mouth-to-mouth resuscitation. First aiders who know CPR really can mean the difference between life and death. But until recently, there wasn't much the victim could do to save himself. Now there is.

It's called "do-it-yourself CPR." Although it is no substitute for immediate medical attention, this first aid tip might keep a heart attack victim conscious long enough to summon help.

Here's how to do it, according to UCLA cardiologist John Michael Criley, M.D., who developed the technique. If you are having a heart attack and begin to lose consciousness, start coughing vigorously—about once every second. Doing so may keep you conscious, possibly until help arrives.

"Coughing causes the muscles of the abdomen and chest to contract in such a way as to keep blood moving to the brain," says Dr. Criley, chief of cardiology at the Harbor UCLA Medical Center. "Our experiments have shown that the technique can maintain blood flow to the brain at levels equal to or greater than a normal heartbeat, and that consciousness can be maintained for a minute and a half, possibly longer."

Even if you don't know CPR, you might be able to save a life by instructing a heart attack victim to keep coughing until help arrives, says Dr. Criley. Symptoms of a heart attack that you should recognize include:

- Dull, but sometimes crushing, pain located toward the center of the chest, possibly extending into the left arm or jaw.
- Shortness of breath.
- Nausea or a cold sweat.
- Faintness.

Remember that do-it-yourself CPR is literally a do-or-die technique to be used *only* if you start to faint or black out. It won't relieve the initial symptoms of a heart attack, nor will it ease the chest pain of angina.

Say Bye-Bye to Back Blows

Up until recently, to unblock a jammed windpipe, you were advised to alternately strike the victim between the shoulder blades and press in and up on the abdomen. You probably recognize the second half of this first aid skill as the Heimlich maneuver. But the first step of this lifesaving dance routine has been abandoned, and with good reason.

"There just isn't any evidence that back blows are any more effective than the Heimlich maneuver," according to Roger D. White, M.D., of the Mayo Clinic Medical School, Rochester, Minnesota, and former chairman of the National Registry of Emergency Medical Technicians. "Airway obstructions are relieved in a majority of cases with just two or three abdominal thrusts."

This being the case, the American Heart Association and the American Red Cross recently dropped the back blows altogether, except in infants under a year old. In their place, they advise trying the Heimlich maneuver.

If the maneuver doesn't work after several attempts, try removing any obvious particles of food or foreign objects from the mouth. Don't probe too deeply. Then try to blow four deep breaths of air into the victim, using mouth-to-mouth resuscitation. If this doesn't work, repeat the cycle.

To do the Heimlich maneuver, stand behind the choking person and reach around the abdomen with both hands. Roll your right hand into a fist, thumb side facing the abdomen. Put your left hand over your right hand. Then squeeze in and up in one motion.

Make certain that you place your hands exactly betweeen the navel and the flexible cartilage at the base of the breastbone. You can feel the cartilage, called the xiphoid process, with your fingers. Squeezing down on the xiphoid may cause internal bleeding, so getting your hands in the right position is very important.

Although back blows have been eliminated for most choking victims, you should still attempt them in infants under a year old, according to Dr. White. A study presented at a national conference on cardiopulmonary resuscitation showed that back blows continue to be an effective way of dislodging foreign objects in infant airways, he says.

Cut and Suck No More

It's a tradition that goes back centuries, but there's been some biting criticism of the practice of slicing into a snakebite and sucking the venom out.

Says pharmacist Susan Shelnutt, assistant director of the Arizona Poison and Drug Information Center in Tucson, "The efficacy of cutting and sucking is seriously in doubt. One, we find that we don't get a lot of poison out when we do that. Two, you can cause more problems, especially if you cut where the skin is not very deep, like the hands and fingers. You can cut through blood vessels or muscles."

Here's what to do instead, according to Shelnutt.

- Keep the victim calm.
- Keep the person from moving too much. Movement hastens the spread of poison through the body.
- Wrap a bandage—1½ to 2 inches wide—around the limb, a few inches above the bite. It should be loose enough, says Shelnutt, for you to be able to slip a finger or two underneath it. If it isn't, loosen it a bit.
- Keep the affected limb lower than the level of the heart.
- Get prompt medical help.

Consider the Tourniquet a Last Resort

Heavy bleeding is about as frightening an emergency as you're likely to see. One way to stem the flow is to apply a tourniquet, but here's a case where one good turn does not deserve another.

The tourniquet is a wide strip of cloth or bandage. It is wrapped around a limb above the wound, then twisted until the bleeding stops. But when you apply a tourniquet, you might cause more damage to blood vessels and nerves than the original injury did. "It's a last resort measure to control bleeding," says C. P. Dail, Jr., a safety instruction associate with the American Red Cross. "You apply a tourniquet to save a life, but when you do so, you expect to lose the limb."

Fortunately, says Dail, such a drastic measure might not be necessary. "Most severe bleeding can be stopped by applying pressure directly on the wound," he says. To apply direct pressure, find a thick piece of clean cloth—a bandage is fine, but a clean towel, sheet, handkerchief or even a T-shirt will do. Place it over the wound and press down with your hand.

If the bleeding continues, try these two steps.

- If an arm or leg is bleeding, raise the limb above the level of the heart. You should do this while continuing to apply direct pressure to the wound.
- While continuing direct pressure on the wound with one hand, apply pressure to a supplying artery with the other. For leg injuries, press with the heel of your hand against the femoral artery, found on the inside surface of the thigh, just below the groin. If the bleeding is in the arm, apply pressure to the brachial artery. To find it, press your fingers against the inside surface of the upper arm, below the armpit.

CHAPTER 37

How to Beat a Bunion

Here's good advice from podiatrists on how to handle this painful foot malady.

A bunion is a painful bump at the base of your big toe that you could do very well without. Its medical name, hallus valgus, means "big toe bent outward." Actually, though, it's the joint at the base of your big toe that's bulging outward. This happens because, due to various structural problems in the foot, the big toe has gradually turned *inward*. The result is an unsightly, calloused, often painful bulge just where you don't need it.

Foot specialists (podiatrists) generally agree that certain preexisting and usually inherited tendencies must be present for a bunion to reach full bloom. Flat feet can be a predisposing factor, for instance. So can a general laxity of the ligaments whose job it is to keep the big toe in place.

Shoes for Bunionnaires

But very often bunions are largely the result of wearing shoes that don't fit. In societies where people go barefoot, bunions are rare. The worst kind of shoes are those that are narrow at the toe and lofty at the heel, because this configuration drives the forefoot into a painfully constricting wedge.

High heels are probably the only reason bunions are more common among women. Still, a pair of snazzy, stiletto-toed Italian loafers can put male feet in the same sort of bind.

For simple, nonsurgical relief for bunions, podiatrists often recommend seeking out the widest, softest shoe you can find. You might even look into special "extra depth" shoes that are wider in the front than the back—one with a toebox measuring a roomy D or E, for example, but a heel with a snug-fitting A or B.

Also, don't be afraid of Dr. Scholl's. Many drugstores carry displays of products to relieve the pain of bunions. Felt or foam "bunion pads," which fit around the bulge, will help distribute shoe pressure more evenly and also reduce irritating friction. Foam "toe spacers," which simply spread the big toe, may also help relieve the pressure.

You might also want to check with a podiatrist about getting fitted for shoe inserts capable of minimizing the structural abnormalities that are at the root of the problem.

The Surgical Alternatives

Really crippling bunions may require surgery. There are more than 100 surgical procedures to correct bunions, ranging from simple removal of the bony prominence to resectioning of the joint, fusion and realignment of the affected toes. Though every case is different, bunion surgery falls into two basic categories.

"Open" bunion surgery requires a two- to four-inch incision along the edge of the foot, so the surgeon can actually *see* the whole area being operated on. In most cases, there's much more involved than simply cutting down the overgrown bone, and this requires an opening large enough for visual inspection. Most bunion surgery can be performed with equal effectiveness by a podiatrist or an orthopedic surgeon and usually requires only local anesthesia. Only rarely is hospitalization required.

After surgery, you may be able to walk home, but that doesn't mean you're home free. Though you may go back to work in a few days or a week, you won't be dancing a jig for at least six weeks. And you may have to wear a fiberglass walking cast for three to six weeks. Bone healing takes six to eight weeks.

"Closed" or "minimal incision" bunion surgery, as its name implies, is performed through a much tinier opening (about ⅛ inch). Guided by feel instead of by sight, the surgeon uses tiny drills similar to those used in dentistry to file off excess bone. He can also reposition bones of the foot, if necessary.

Minimal incision foot surgery is still the subject of considerable medical controversy. "It is impossible to correct the functioning of the foot through such a small incision," contends Harold Vogler, D.P.M., professor and chairman of the Department of Surgery at the Pennsylvania College of Podiatric Medicine. "There are some nice results from minimal incision surgery, but it is unpredictable and therefore we at the Department of Surgery do not recommend it for bunions."

"A bunion deformity is usually two things: enlargement and displacement," adds Dalton McGlamry, D.P.M., past president of the American Podiatry Association. "If you have only the enlargement and not a major displacement, the quick surgery is fine. Unfortunately, over 95 percent of all bunions involve some degree of displacement and much more serious problems."

Other foot surgeons maintain that minimal incision surgery causes less pain and less trauma to bone and tissue and results in quicker recovery. If you're unsure which alternative to choose, discuss both with your podiatrist. And try to find a surgeon who's trained in both procedures, suggests Thomas DeLauro, vice-president and academic dean of the New York College of Podiatric Medicine.

CHAPTER 38

The Pros and Cons of Bargain Eyeglasses

Buying nonprescription spectacles over the counter can make sense, but only if you know what shape your eyes are in before you walk into the store.

There is a variety of bargain spectacles to be had over the counter at a fraction of the cost of prescription eyewear. But are they worth even the low price you pay, and will they do the job or harm your already impaired vision?

It depends.

"A problem occurs when people need glasses, usually for reading, and make their own diagnosis without having an eye exam by an optometrist or ophthalmologist," says Robert Yolton, O.D., Ph.D., associate professor of psychophysiology at the Pacific University College of Optometry in Forest Grove, Oregon. "They could have the beginnings of severe problems that, if not corrected, could lead to total loss of sight or even loss of life." Ophthalmologist Louis Wilson, M.D., of Emory University Medical Center, Atlanta, concurs. "I usually have no objection to over-the-counter glasses if the person has had a thorough exam. In fact, I've recommended these glasses to patients, and they are usually surprised to hear a doctor suggest they buy eyeglasses at a dime store or bargain house."

Eyewear Options Aplenty

Spectacles were once crude, ugly, unscientific magnifiers, usually spurned by physicians and sold by ragged peddlers in market squares.

Today, people looking to place a matched pair of lenses before their needy eyes find a supermarketful of more appealing options—glass, plastic and tinted lenses, bifocals and trifocals and an endless array of frames. They also find that prescription eyeglasses cost several times more than off-the-rack reading specs. This price differential can be eye-opening to those on a tight budget.

"A lot of people over 40 can see at a distance but have trouble reading, so they buy over-the-counter glasses for part-time use. But they should keep in mind the old saying that you get what you pay for," says Dr. Yolton. "These glasses are mass-produced and work in some cases, but aren't designed to handle certain eye conditions."

Blurred near vision affects almost everyone over age 40 and is often traced to presbyopia, a minor focusing problem that hampers reading and other close work. But many people in that age group also have astigmatism, a condition where the cornea is shaped like half a football, instead of being round like a basketball. To correct the problem, the wearer needs custom-made lenses, not bargain eyeglasses.

Also, for good vision, the pupil of the eye must line up with the center of the lens. Most over-the-counter eyewear is made to general standards, which means the alignment may be off. "If this occurs, things can look clear and in focus, but the wearer can get headaches, tired eyes or other eyestrain symptoms," says Dr. Yolton.

Risk Reduction

The real risk, though, is that the cost-conscious buyer won't have a thorough examination that could point to a serious eye condition. Glaucoma, for instance, can go unnoticed without proper testing because the loss of sight is so gradual. By the time you realize there's a problem, much of the damage is irreversible, and peripheral vision can be lost. With glaucoma, pressure builds in the eye and kills the nerves that send messages to the brain. People over age 40 are highly susceptible and should have their eyes checked at least every two years.

An examination can also spot hypertension brewing. Leaking blood vessels in the eye are usually good indicators of high blood pressure. Early detection can prevent more severe problems.

Exams are crucial for diabetics, says Dr. Wilson. For some unknown reason, the diabetic body grows new, fragile blood vessels in the center and rear of the eyes. "A routine exam is important because these vessels can break. Vision can be impaired and scar tissue forms. If caught in time, the vessels can be sealed with laser therapy."

More Than Aesthetics

If you've had an exam and been cleared for a pair of off-the-rack eyeglasses, there's more to consider than merely how they look on your face.

The specs generally come in about ten different powers. The lower the number, the less the magnification. "Another advantage of having an exam is that you'll know which power you need, and you won't have to guess when you get to the store," says Dr. Wilson.

Look for tempered lenses because they meet federal standards about breakage, says Don Schuman, O.D., an eyeglass-design specialist also at the Pacific University College of Optometry. "Check to see how the lenses are mounted. The edges of prescription lenses are ground into a V-shape to fit securely into a groove in the frame. The cheaper glasses usually aren't constructed with as well designed a groove, which means a blow to the face could more easily pop the lenses out and into the eye."

Lenses should be checked for flaws, says Dr. Schuman. "Look through them carefully, because they are mass-produced and can have imperfections that can distort or blur your vision."

To do this, Dr. Schuman suggests putting on the glasses and looking at a horizontal or vertical line. While turning your head, view the line from all different angles through the lenses. Does the line ripple? If it does, the lenses are of poor quality. Try on a different pair and test them, too.

Be aware also that many people need a different lens prescription for each eye, whereas with bargain glasses the magnification is the same in both lenses.

Over-the-counter frames won't be adjusted like prescription frames, so comfort and fit should be checked carefully. "One ear is higher than the other on some people, so the frames may sit on your face at an angle, which can be irritating or cause headaches. Also, the nose bridge on cheaper frames is usually a standard size, so the glasses may slide down or sit too high," says Dr. Schuman. "In either case, the field of vision can be hampered."

Residents of some states, including Louisiana, Kansas, Massachusetts, Minnesota, New York and Rhode Island, need not ponder whether to go with over-the-counter glasses, because state laws prohibit their sale. Elsewhere, consumers are on their own.

"There's nothing dastardly about these glasses, and I don't think anyone's out to swindle or deceive the public," says Dr. Yolton. "But be sure you have your eyes examined thoroughly and regularly by an optometrist or ophthalmologist. If over-the-counter glasses are recommended and they work for you, they may be all you need."

CHAPTER 39

The Experts' Guide to Healthier Gums and Teeth

Four dental professionals answer your questions about what causes—and fights—cavities and gum disease.

It's what you don't know about dental problems that hurts you. Here is the lowdown on plaque (one of the leading causes of infection in the United States), gum disease and other dental menaces from four top experts from around the country.

Q. *What is plaque?*

A. Plaque is the name given to the bacteria that literally colonize your mouth. Even the cleanest, healthiest mouth harbors a community of 330 different identified species of bacteria, linked in what Kenneth S. Kornman, D.D.S., Ph.D., chairman of the Department of Periodontics of the University of Texas Health Science Center, calls "one of the most complex bacterial ecosystems in the body." They all live quite happily together, actually keeping each other "in check," says Susan Karabin, D.D.S., assistant clinical professor of periodontics at Columbia University. (Some scientists even suspect that *Streptococcus* bacteria control the growth of several microorganisms that cause gum disease infection.) Their relationship, however, is in a delicate balance. When one becomes prominent, it throws off those checks and balances that keep your mouth healthy, and that's when you get cavities and gum disease.

Q. *Can I actually see the plaque on my teeth?*

A. In a healthy mouth, plaque is a thin, invisible film of bacterial colonies that are only about 1 to 20 cells thick. It becomes more visible when the colonies begin to multiply, which is what happens when you don't clean your teeth regularly. Then it may look like a white, sticky film, although it should not be confused with food debris. "If it's your peanut-butter-and-jelly sandwich, it's not plaque," says Dr. Kornman. It becomes quite visible when it combines with calcium and phosphorus in the mouth and hardens, forming a barnaclelike substance called tartar, or calculus. That's what your dentist or dental hygienist has to chip and scrape from your teeth.

Q. *Is all plaque the same?*

A. No. There is a considerable difference between the plaque that grows above the gum line and that which grows below it. Above the gum line, on the part of the teeth you can see, the plaque is aerobic, meaning it needs oxygen to survive. It also needs to be fed regularly, and unfortunately, it enjoys the high-sugar, high-carbohydrate American diet. It uses the sucrose to form a sticky substance that helps it adhere to the tooth surface, where it acid-drills into tooth enamel, causing cavities. Scientists believe they have identified the particular bacterium that causes dental cavities, one called *Streptococcus mutans.*

Q. *What about the bacteria growing beneath the gums?*

A. Below the gum line, it's another story. The bacteria there are anaerobic, meaning that they don't need oxygen. And they don't need to share your meals. They feed instead on what they can, usually the protein from your gum tissue. Scientists don't know which of the microorganisms below your gums can cause gum disease—the leading cause of tooth loss in the United States—although they have narrowed the list to six or seven likely culprits. They do know it's likely to be more than one doing you harm.

Q. *So is all plaque harmful?*

A. Not at all. "You never want to have a sterile mouth," says Michael G. Newman, D.D.S., professor in the section of periodontics at the University of California at Los Angeles. In fact, every mucous membrane of the body is lined with bacteria. "That is part of the defense mechanism that developed for your body," says Dr. Kornman. "They're protective. But their presence in some cases may not only be protective. It may also be destructive."

Q. *When does it stop helping me and start hurting me?*
A. With a lack of thorough and consistent oral hygiene, you allow a bacterial population explosion to take place in your mouth. Often, the protective bacteria are crowded out by microorganisms with less benign intentions. The environment of your mouth changes. And, like a neighborhood where one unsavory character settles, it attracts others and, eventually, "there goes the neighborhood."

Q. *How long does this population explosion take?*
A. Minutes after your dentist has thoroughly cleaned your teeth, the bacterial colonies begin to grow again, but it is 24 to 48 hours before the harmful bacteria—the ones that creep into the crevices between your gums and teeth and cause infection—start to flourish again. By then, they may even have caused some gum damage, says Dr. Kornman.

Q. *It sounds like they grow on different time schedules. Do they?*
A. They do. The earliest colonizers of your mouth are the germs known as *Streptococcus* and *Actinomyces*. "Most of them are the healthy bugs," says Dr. Newman. If you don't clean your teeth, the colonies grow and the bacterial population changes. In one research study in which healthy volunteers didn't brush for three weeks, the *Streptococcus* population started to dwindle as the *Actinomyces* grew larger. The volunteers wound up with thicker plaque and/or gingivitis, a condition that is characterized by tender, red, bleeding gums and is often the precursor of gum disease. Over time, new bacteria join the crowd, attracted by other bacteria and the changing environment of the increasingly unhygienic mouth. "There are certain bac-

bone and tissue is destroyed as it "retreats from the advancing front of the infection," says Dr. Newman.

Q. *It sounds horrible. If I don't take care of my teeth and let ie harmful bacteria invade my gums, am I doomed to losing eth?*

A. No. Treatment of gum disease is usually quite suc- sful. It may be limited to scaling and root planing— noving deposits from the deep gum pockets where they ect. It may involve something called a periodontal flap edure, whereby gum tissue is moved away from the n and the bones and the entire area is cleaned out. etimes the disease responds well to antibiotics. But ts caution that these treatments are not a cure. Bone irreversible, and once you have had the disease, you n susceptible. "And surgery doesn't really do any- out provide for the patient a starting ground for a nance program," says Dr. Löe. You have the ibility of keeping your mouth clean. Preventing ease is far easier and far more pleasant than treat-

some people more susceptible to plaque buildup s?

and that's the curious thing about plaque. It ffect each person differently, and it may be quite t different sites in the same mouth. Oddly u may have periodontal disease affecting only a your mouth. Scientists refer to gum disease as nist" ailment. The makings of the disease— bacteria—may be in your mouth or nearby at ply waiting for the right conditions to sprout. t weakens the immune system—poor nutri- l health, use of broad-spectrum antibiotics, eatments—may make your mouth ripe for Any increase—or decrease—in the popula- these microorganisms may also invite the a to run rampant, as can improper hygiene. people in particular who are very suscepti- se.

teria that live off the by-products of other bacteria and have a kind of parasitic relationship with them," explains Dr. Kornman. This stratified growth of oral bacteria is called bacterial succession, and the last bacterium that takes hold tends to do the most damage.

Q. *Is there a good way to keep this population explosion from occurring in the first place?*

A. Prevention is the key word here. If you keep plaque down to a minimum (it's impossible to remove it entirely, says Dr. Kornman), you won't set the stage for this dangerous bacterial bloom. At the same time, you'll also be cutting down on cavities because you'll be brushing away both the germs and the sugary food they eat. At the very minimum, you need to brush at least twice a day, floss to remove food debris and plaque from between teeth and have regular dental checkups so your dentist can remove tartar and any plaque that's crept below the gum line.

Q. *Are there any recommended ways to brush and floss?*

A. That's a good point. "Plaque removal is not accomplished with 15 seconds of tasting a toothpaste," says Harald Löe, D.D.S., Dr.Odont., director of the National Institute of Dental Research in Bethesda, Maryland. Some people, Dr. Karabin notes, "brush and brush and brush and don't even touch the plaque." The recommended technique is to hold your brush at a slant—roughly a 45-degree angle—and brush at the gum margin with gentle, short, scrubbing strokes on both sides of the teeth. To floss, take a strand of waxed or unwaxed floss and wrap it around the tooth, rubbing it up and down. "The seesaw method doesn't usually touch plaque," warns Dr. Karabin. To see how well you're doing, use a disclosing tablet or mouthwash, which stains the plaque. (It is water-soluble, so the stain can be brushed away.)

Q. *Should I be using any of the antiplaque toothpastes or mouthwashes?*

A. As long as you don't have gum disease, some of the products that claim to reduce plaque or tartar may be somewhat effective as an adjunct to regular, basic care. Products that contain essential oils, pyrophosphates and even baking soda and peroxide have been shown in some tests to do what they claim to do. But the experts issue an important warning: These products can only prevent plaque growth and prevent tartar. They don't reach bacteria under the gums nor do they cure gum disease or gingivitis. Also, plaque affects each person differently. "Plaque reduction of 60 percent may prevent gingivitis for you but may do nothing for me," says Dr. Kornman.

Q. *Is there anything that works well?*

A. Yes, a substance called chlorhexidene, which is an antimicrobial. It actually reverses gingivitis. It was first used to fight plaque and treat gingivitis in Europe and Canada. The U.S. Food and Drug Administration has approved chlorhexidene as a mouth rinse, but it is available only by prescription. Its only drawbacks are its bitter taste and the staining, which is not permanent, that occurs with frequent use.

Q. *I've seen metal dental picks for removing tartar—just like the ones my dentist uses—available in my local drugstore. Are they effective?*

A. "The best thing I can tell you is that I took one home and my wife used it and fractured a tooth," says Dr. Kornman. "I would not advise that these be used for two reasons. First, they're sharp and can damage gum tissue and teeth. Second, they sit around uncleaned and may even spread germs to the mouth."

Q. *If I remove plaque faithfully every day, is there any reason that I have to see my dentist every year?*

A. The dentist is the only one who can tell you how well you're removing plaque. He or she will examine your teeth for cavities and, using a periodontal probe, will explore the space beneath your gums to determine how deep the pockets are where the plaque collects. He or she can also determine whether there has been any bone or gum deterioration by taking x-rays. You need to know if you have plaque

under the gums because home care simply
then.

Q. *How often do I have to see my dentist*

A. That depends on whether you have
annual checkup is fine for detecting ca
have a history of gum disease, you sh
every three to four months, says Dr. K

Q. *Gum disease sounds serious. Is it*

A. Gum disease, or periodontal
most frequently occurring infection
By some estimates, three-quarters
in some form, usually as ging
(though not always) leads to fu
ease. It is, of course, a bacterial
destroys soft gum tissue and b
periodontal disease causes tee
frightening thing about perio
silent epidemic," says Dr. N
preceded by red, tender, bl
ease can be relatively sym

Q. *How does it lead to*

A. It leads to tooth
scientists still don't com
still unidentified—cau
body to turn on the i
of gingivitis, the red
tem—part of your
you fight off the d
vanced gum dise
gums or betweer
then something
against you. "I
stroying the l
much of the d
battle betwe
with the im
Researcher

Q. *Who are they?*

A. People who've already had gum disease. People who have crooked teeth—simply because it's difficult to clean the teeth properly. Diabetics also tend to get gum disease at an early age, and it can make their diabetes more difficult to control, says Dr. Kornman. Likewise, if their diabetes is out of control, the gum disease gets worse. About half of all pregnant women suffer from something called pregnancy gingivitis, which usually hits in the second trimester when there are hormonal changes in their serum and gum fluid. "The fluid contains high levels of estrogen, and there are certain bacteria that love that and grow on it," says Dr. Karabin. Pregnant women need to clean their teeth meticulously during that time, and some may even need to see their dentist monthly so the disease doesn't advance. There are also some people who get periodontal disease at a very early age—as young as three. Researchers suspect a minor genetic flaw that affects white blood cells, which are part of the immune system. Others think there may be a familial connection.

Q. *You mean they catch it from their family?*

A. Exactly. Like many infections, periodontal disease can be "catching." You can even transmit plaque bacteria through "mouth-to-mouth contamination." "We know a major implantation of *Streptococcus mutans,* which is responsible for tooth decay, occurs in a transfer from mother to child, which is one of the important routes of establishing an infection in newborns," says Dr. Löe. You can pass plaque bacteria to someone by sharing a utensil or a toothbrush.

Q. *Is there any nutritional advice I can follow to help fight off a plaque attack?*

A. Most experts advise eating a good, balanced diet to help you keep up your general health. "Your general health is always reflected in your mouth," says Dr. Karabin. "Your ability to fight off infection—your immunological system—is directly affected by your health." Some experts recommend either taking a vitamin C supplement or increasing intake of foods rich in vitamin C, because C helps in the production of collagen in the gum tissues. "This may be important only in the elderly, who may not get enough vitamin C," suggests Dr. Löe. Specifically, to help fight tooth decay, cut down on sugars and other carbohydrates that feed *Streptococcus mutans.* The bug that causes cavities uses sugars to form a sticky glue that adheres to the teeth, and it excretes acids and toxins that bore through tooth enamel. And remember, germs don't care where the sugar comes from. The sugar from a candy bar and the sugar from a peach is all the same to them. It helps to brush or rinse after any kind of high-sugar meal.

CHAPTER 40

Battling the Allergy Dust Bug

This microscopic monster is a menace you can tame.

If you're part of the vast majority that doesn't live where the relative humidity is always low, you should know that you're sharing your quarters with a colony of creatures straight out of a Saturday matinee bug-eyed monster movie.

They're uglier than Godzilla, harder to get rid of than Dracula and more frightening-looking than the thing from *Alien,* and they have less manners than King Kong.

They're dust mites, and they're probably in your home, no matter how hospital-clean it may appear. That's because they're in almost everybody's home—one study reports finding dust mites in 99 of 100 homes tested in the Baltimore area.

But you wouldn't know it, because these hideous horrors of allergy are so small you can't even see them. They're so tiny, says the American College of Allergists, that thousands of the little buggers have been counted in a single gram of house dust.

But their small size doesn't prevent them from having a heavyweight impact on your allergies. Dust mites—actually their feces—are the single most common foreign protein that people inhale in their homes.

We Provide the Food

"It's unfortunate that people don't learn about mites in school," explains Thomas Platts-Mills, M.D., Ph.D., a professor of medicine in the Division of Allergy at the University of Virginia Medical School. "There's an absolute gap in public knowledge about these species that exist between small insects and bacteria.

"House dust mites are very close relatives to the mites that burrow into people's skin and cause scabies, but these household mites are not parasites. They're scavengers, eating the skin flakes, or dander, that we shed all the time. You can't deny them this food—skin shedding is a natural human process, and there's no way to prevent it."

They're Not House-Trained!

Luckily, Dr. Platts-Mills says, our lungs are not full of nasty little live mites.

"They don't get inhaled because they have tremendously sticky feet that hold them onto surfaces like rugs and other fabric. Vacuuming, in fact, only removes the dead ones.

"What we mostly inhale—and become allergic to—is their feces. Some people are allergic to the proteins in their body parts, but 80 percent of those who develop symptoms are reacting to the feces alone. And there's a lot to react to. They breed quickly and each mite eats enough to produce at least ten fecal pellets a day.

"These pellets are remarkable—they're so light they stay in the air for a good ten minutes after they're disturbed, and the membrane that covers the outside of the pellet is so strong that you could soak it in salt water for 16 hours without harming it in the least."

That's especially bad news. It means that the pellets don't break down very quickly. They keep their allergy-causing potential for months, and just moving a pillow or walking across a carpet is enough to stir them up into the air.

Dr. Platts-Mills feels that this constant exposure is the reason that an astonishing 10 to 15 percent of the general population has developed an allergy to these unwelcome guests. Among asthmatics and people with multiple allergies, the figure rises to around 40 percent.

Are these creatures unbeatable—are their feces indestructible? Are we all doomed to suffer sneezing, sniffles and the personal degradation of inhaling endless amounts of minuscule mite excrement?

Did Tokyo Give Up to Godzilla?

Of course not! Think back to those Saturday matinee solutions. When Godzilla took down one high-tension wire too many, they bleached his bones with an oxygen bomb! When King Kong made an even bigger mess of New York than usual, they sent airplanes to show him the shortcut down to Fifth Avenue!

The elimination of your mite population is even easier. "They can't survive when the relative humidity is less than 50 percent," Dr. Platts-Mills says.

"Controlling humidity is the single most important factor," agrees Richard Weber, M.D., chief of the Allergy-Immunology Division at Fitzsimmons Army Medical Center. "Air conditioning is very good for reducing humidity,

teria that live off the by-products of other bacteria and have a kind of parasitic relationship with them," explains Dr. Kornman. This stratified growth of oral bacteria is called bacterial succession, and the last bacterium that takes hold tends to do the most damage.

Q. *Is there a good way to keep this population explosion from occurring in the first place?*

A. Prevention is the key word here. If you keep plaque down to a minimum (it's impossible to remove it entirely, says Dr. Kornman), you won't set the stage for this dangerous bacterial bloom. At the same time, you'll also be cutting down on cavities because you'll be brushing away both the germs and the sugary food they eat. At the very minimum, you need to brush at least twice a day, floss to remove food debris and plaque from between teeth and have regular dental checkups so your dentist can remove tartar and any plaque that's crept below the gum line.

Q. *Are there any recommended ways to brush and floss?*

A. That's a good point. "Plaque removal is not accomplished with 15 seconds of tasting a toothpaste," says Harald Löe, D.D.S., Dr.Odont., director of the National Institute of Dental Research in Bethesda, Maryland. Some people, Dr. Karabin notes, "brush and brush and brush and don't even touch the plaque." The recommended technique is to hold your brush at a slant—roughly a 45-degree angle—and brush at the gum margin with gentle, short, scrubbing strokes on both sides of the teeth. To floss, take a strand of waxed or unwaxed floss and wrap it around the tooth, rubbing it up and down. "The seesaw method doesn't usually touch plaque," warns Dr. Karabin. To see how well you're doing, use a disclosing tablet or mouthwash, which stains the plaque. (It is water-soluble, so the stain can be brushed away.)

Q. *Should I be using any of the antiplaque toothpastes or mouthwashes?*

A. As long as you don't have gum disease, some of the products that claim to reduce plaque or tartar may be somewhat effective as an adjunct to regular, basic care. Products that contain essential oils, pyrophosphates and even baking soda and peroxide have been shown in some tests to do what they claim to do. But the experts issue an important warning: These products can only prevent plaque growth and prevent tartar. They don't reach bacteria under the gums nor do they cure gum disease or gingivitis. Also, plaque affects each person differently. "Plaque reduction of 60 percent may prevent gingivitis for you but may do nothing for me," says Dr. Kornman.

Q. *Is there anything that works well?*

A. Yes, a substance called chlorhexidene, which is an antimicrobial. It actually reverses gingivitis. It was first used to fight plaque and treat gingivitis in Europe and Canada. The U.S. Food and Drug Administration has approved chlorhexidene as a mouth rinse, but it is available only by prescription. Its only drawbacks are its bitter taste and the staining, which is not permanent, that occurs with frequent use.

Q. *I've seen metal dental picks for removing tartar—just like the ones my dentist uses—available in my local drugstore. Are they effective?*

A. "The best thing I can tell you is that I took one home and my wife used it and fractured a tooth," says Dr. Kornman. "I would not advise that these be used for two reasons. First, they're sharp and can damage gum tissue and teeth. Second, they sit around uncleaned and may even spread germs to the mouth."

Q. *If I remove plaque faithfully every day, is there any reason that I have to see my dentist every year?*

A. The dentist is the only one who can tell you how well you're removing plaque. He or she will examine your teeth for cavities and, using a periodontal probe, will explore the space beneath your gums to determine how deep the pockets are where the plaque collects. He or she can also determine whether there has been any bone or gum deterioration by taking x-rays. You need to know if you have plaque under the gums because home care simply doesn't work then.

Q. *How often do I have to see my dentist?*

A. That depends on whether you have gum disease. An annual checkup is fine for detecting cavities, but if you have a history of gum disease, you should be evaluated every three to four months, says Dr. Kornman.

Q. *Gum disease sounds serious. Is it?*

A. Gum disease, or periodontal disease, is one of the most frequently occurring infections in the United States. By some estimates, three-quarters of the population has it in some form, usually as gingivitis, which frequently (though not always) leads to full-blown periodontal disease. It is, of course, a bacterial infection that attacks and destroys soft gum tissue and bone. If left to run its course, periodontal disease causes teeth to loosen and fall out. The frightening thing about periodontal disease is that it is "the silent epidemic," says Dr. Newman. Although frequently preceded by red, tender, bleeding gums, periodontal disease can be relatively symptomless.

Q. *How does it lead to tooth loss?*

A. It leads to tooth loss in a very peculiar way that scientists still don't completely understand. The bacteria—still unidentified—cause an infection. This stimulates the body to turn on the immune system to fight it. In the case of gingivitis, the red gums represent the inflammatory system—part of your immune function—kicking in to help you fight off the disease. In fact, one of the signs of advanced gum disease is pus that erupts from beneath the gums or between the teeth when the gum is pressed. But then something more happens. Your immune system turns against you. "Part of this immune response ends up destroying the local tissue," explains Dr. Kornman. In fact, much of the destruction of bone and tissue is a result of this battle between infection and your own immune system, with the immune system inflicting much of the damage. Researchers theorize—they're not sure—that some of the bone and tissue is destroyed as it "retreats from the advancing front of the infection," says Dr. Newman.

Q. *It sounds horrible. If I don't take care of my teeth and let the harmful bacteria invade my gums, am I doomed to losing teeth?*

A. No. Treatment of gum disease is usually quite successful. It may be limited to scaling and root planing—removing deposits from the deep gum pockets where they collect. It may involve something called a periodontal flap procedure, whereby gum tissue is moved away from the tooth and the bones and the entire area is cleaned out. Sometimes the disease responds well to antibiotics. But experts caution that these treatments are not a cure. Bone loss is irreversible, and once you have had the disease, you remain susceptible. "And surgery doesn't really do anything but provide for the patient a starting ground for a maintenance program," says Dr. Löe. You have the responsibility of keeping your mouth clean. Preventing gum disease is far easier and far more pleasant than treatment.

Q. *Are some people more susceptible to plaque buildup than others?*

A. Yes, and that's the curious thing about plaque. It seems to affect each person differently, and it may be quite different at different sites in the same mouth. Oddly enough, you may have periodontal disease affecting only a few teeth in your mouth. Scientists refer to gum disease as an "opportunist" ailment. The makings of the disease—the harmful bacteria—may be in your mouth or nearby at all times, simply waiting for the right conditions to sprout. Anything that weakens the immune system—poor nutrition or general health, use of broad-spectrum antibiotics, some cancer treatments—may make your mouth ripe for this infection. Any increase—or decrease—in the population of one of these microorganisms may also invite the harmful bacteria to run rampant, as can improper hygiene. There are some people in particular who are very susceptible to gum disease.

but people in very warm and moist climates may also need a dehumidifier or two in the house. Be careful to empty any standing pools of water in these units regularly."

For getting dead mites and their fecal pellets out of your house, Dr. Platts-Mills recommends specialized vacuum cleaners that don't blow lots of tiny particles back into the room.

"Some of these machines run the dirt through a water chamber and others have a superfine filter. But no matter how fine the filter, people with any kind of dust allergies should always wear a mask when vacuuming.

"You can even get live mites out of your bedding if you keep in mind that neither cool washing nor detergents harms them. Hot washing, however, will destroy them."

Get the Bugs out of Your Bed

"The mite count is almost always highest in the bedroom," adds Dr. Weber. "It's the best room in the house not to have carpeting. Studies have proven that dust control measures such as encasing mattresses in plastic really help. Encasing is very easy to do—you can buy plastic cases ready-made, or just use sheets of plastic sealed with tape to wrap the mattress like a Christmas present.

"Get rid of feather pillows and down comforters, too," he recommends. He feels that many people who think they're allergic to feathers are actually reacting to the mites in the pillows. He recommends pillows stuffed with Dacron or other synthetic materials.

The Carpet Connection

"Deep-pile shag carpets," says Dr. Weber, "are absolutely hopeless when it comes to mite removal. The best flooring for moist climates is hardwood or linoleum, but even short-pile carpet is better than deep pile."

Dr. Weber agrees that "vacuuming is very effective at getting the problem into the air. Unquestionably, you really stir up the stuff when you vacuum, so clean with a damp mop or cloth whenever possible.

"Mites are especially fond of furniture as well. You should definitely avoid upholstery with deep, sculpted fabric. Hardwood and cane furniture is best, followed by 'nonfabrics' like vinyl, leather and Naugahyde."

The Worst Time Is Summer

"Mite colonies, which thrive at 70 percent relative humidity, tend to hit their peak in late summer, around August and September," explains Dr. Weber. "When the home heating system comes on, their numbers drop off. The colonies hit their lowest point in January and start to rise again in spring when the heat goes off and the humidity goes up."

That makes winter a perfect time to implement a mite control program. Consider getting the carpet out of the bedroom, encasing the mattress and maybe even trading in the old fabric sofa in the family room.

Then, when spring arrives, be ready with the air conditioning and/or dehumidifiers. Dr. Weber suggests that you can buy indoor thermometers that also show the humidity so you can check the level in your home. One summer of low humidity will make you feel great, extend the life of your home and kill lots of mites.

CHAPTER 41

A Parent's Guide to Childhood Emergencies

Here's the practical help you need to handle almost any situation.

Kids have boundless curiosity—it's part of being young, after all. But that insatiable desire to "get into everything" also makes them exceptionally vulnerable to catastrophe. Learning to climb a ladder, for example, or open the cap on a bottle are sure signs that your child's motor skills are developing normally. But those achievements are also fraught with danger. It's little wonder that trauma—serious injury—is the leading cause of death in children. In fact, it's been called "the last major plague of the young."

Short of locking your child in a foam rubber chest until he's 18, there's nothing you can do to guarantee his safety all the time. For those occasions when your preventive measures fall short, you must be prepared to manage life's little—and not so little—emergencies.

Knowing When to Get Help

When can you treat your child at home, and when do you call the pediatrician or head for the emergency room of your local hospital?

"Probably that's the most difficult question for a parent to answer," says Gary Fleisher, M.D., medical director of the emergency department of Children's Hospital, Boston. "It depends on whether it's an accident or an illness. For the young infant under three months of age, any signs of illness—fever, irritability or lethargy—should be checked by a physician. Many times for an older child, with the onset of illness, the parents can treat the disorder at home after contacting a physician. I think the complaints or symptoms that would bring kids into the emergency room would be unusually high fever, unusual sleepiness or drowsiness, if the child appears to be drinking less than usual—a sign of dehydration—unusual rash and any difficulty breathing."

Your Reaction Matters

Let's face it: A trip to the emergency room is no fun. But there's much that you and the doctors and nurses treating your child can do to ease the pain.

Stay calm. "Basically, what we try to do is persuade the parent to maintain as calm an atmosphere as possible, because children sense the fear," says Laura Rhodes, nurse manager of the emergency center at St. Luke's and Texas Children's Center in Houston. "We try to let them stay with the child as much as possible. We try to give them the information they need. Lots of times, people feel better if they have information, even if they can't sort it all out."

Be honest. Answer children's questions as truthfully as possible. Even if they're too young to understand, talking children through an emergency can ease the tension, if not the pain.

"Parents should reassure their kids by talking to them, touching or stroking them—whatever methods they have used at home—to make them feel more secure," Rhodes says.

For infants, adds Dr. Fleisher, it is important to keep them warm and comfortable, to feed them if they are hungry. At the other end of the pediatric scale—teenagers—the main thing is to treat them as adults. "You can simplify things a little bit," he says, "but you want to get them involved in the process and have them feel they're in control."

Try to be patient. "My son, who's six, had some sutures on his chin," says Dr. Fleisher. "I brought him in and one of my colleagues stitched him up. I held him, it hurt him, and he cried. When I got him home—it was right after Halloween—he said to me, 'Daddy, I want you to go into my bag of candy and take one of the chocolate kisses, 'cause you gave me comfort when I had my stitches.' At the time, you would have thought I was killing him!

"The point is, even if you apparently fail, and your child is still screaming and crying and hard to deal with, I think that at some level you've done some good. It can never hurt to be kind."

Be Prepared

Knowing what to do in an emergency can ease your child's pain and your anxiety. It helps to keep emergency telephone numbers and first aid supplies handy. First aid training may be helpful, too.

For many childhood emergencies, there are some basic skills you should know. Here are some practical first aid tips for injuries that may occur along your child's sometimes rocky road.

Bee sting. When you were a kid, maybe your mom used mud or baking soda to "draw out" the bee's business end. Sorry, Mom, but that's not the best way. Instead, just gently scrape the stinger and the insect's venom sac out of the skin. To keep swelling down, cover the area with an ice bag. Watch for signs of allergic shock, including muscle cramps, tightness in the chest and difficulty breathing. If you notice any of these signs, seek emergency assistance immediately. An allergic reaction to an insect sting can be life-threatening.

Bicycle fork injury. If your child crushes her foot or leg between the bicycle fork and the spokes of her bicycle, the injuries very well could go beyond mere first aid measures. A torn skin flap, for example, could require plastic surgery. It is best to consult your physician or go to the emergency room of your local hospital.

Bloody nose. Forget tilting your child's head back or applying ice to the bridge of his nose, says Dr. Fleisher. "If you feel your own nose, you'll find the part that's next to your face is bony, and the part that's down at the tip is soft. The part that bleeds is the soft part. All you have to do is squeeze it to stop the bleeding."

Broken bones. Unless you have specific training in the emergency treatment of broken bones, leave them alone. Unless the child is in immediate danger—say, in a burning car or lying on the railroad tracks with a freight train bearing down on him—don't move him or let him move. Call for emergency assistance right away.

Bruises. Use ice or cold cloths to keep the swelling down. Serious bruises, or contusions, may require more than first aid.

The Well-Stocked First Aid Kit

What your first aid kit contains depends on where you plan to use it. Unless you live next door to Billy's Reptile Farm, for example, you probably don't need a snakebite kit.

Here, according to the American Red Cross, are some basic supplies your kit ought to include.

- Adhesive bandages, in assorted sizes.
- Adhesive tape.
- Sterile gauze pads in assorted sizes, the larger the better.
- Gauze roller bandage.
- Large dressings—18×36 and 24×32 inches.
- Triangular bandages.
- Scissors.
- Tweezers.

Should you include first aid creams or ointments? According to the Red Cross, they aren't necessary. Clean water is the only substance that should be used

Bump on the head. If it's just a small injury, follow the procedure for bruises. If it seems to be more serious than that, consult your physician. If the skin is broken, don't attempt to cleanse it and don't put any first aid ointments, sprays or creams on it. If the skull is fractured underneath, you could cause more serious damage. It goes without saying (or ought to) that any loss of consciousness, slurred speech or other serious symptoms require advanced and immediate emergency medical care.

Burns and scalds. For minor burns, the best "treatment" is cool water. Burns with redness and swelling require up to two hours under the faucet or in a sinkful of cold water.

on a deep wound. Triple antibiotic ointments are beneficial, though, for minor cuts and scrapes.

Many pediatricians recommend that you keep some syrup of ipecac on hand. That's to induce vomiting in cases of poisoning. However, be sure to check with your doctor or local poison control center before giving a poison victim anything by mouth.

What about over-the-counter drugs, like aspirin, acetaminophen, antacids or antihistamines? As a practical matter, says Gary Fleisher, M.D., medical director of the emergency department of Children's Hospital, Boston, these medicines are probably already in your medicine cabinet, and they really aren't designed for emergency use. An antihistamine tablet, for example, isn't really strong enough to counter a serious allergic reaction to a bee sting.

Some people find it useful to keep emergency supplies in a handy carryall such as a small fishing tackle box. That way, they can carry what they need to the injured child instead of the other way around.

Obviously, first aid supplies won't be enough for very serious injuries. But they are useful for the everyday bumps and scrapes of childhood.

Don't use ice. And do not use ointments, sprays, butter or other home remedies.

Major burn injuries—charred skin with heavy tissue destruction—are best handled by medical professionals. Don't do anything or put anything on the burn. Seek immediate medical assistance.

Choking. Inhaling food or foreign objects is a leading cause of accidental death in infancy, often during the first four to eight weeks of life. Depending on the child's age, you may administer back blows, abdominal thrusts, or both.

Convulsions. Here's a case that best illustrates one of the aims of first aid: cause no further harm. Don't allow the child to hurt himself. Clear the area of furniture around the child while he's convulsing. Don't try to hold him down. Don't try to put anything in his mouth. Don't immerse him in water. *Do* seek medical help immediately.

Cuts. For minor cuts, gently clean with soap and water and cover with a sterile dressing. For more serious wounds, apply pressure over the site with a thick dressing—a clean cloth or handkerchief will do, or even your hand if there's nothing else available. If possible, elevate the injured part above the level of the heart. Seek emergency assistance as soon as possible.

Dental injuries. If your child should lose a tooth as a result of injuries, the American Association of Endodontists recommends the following steps. First, find the missing tooth. Then pick up the tooth by the crown (the white part), not by its root, and place it back in its socket. Failing that, put the tooth between the child's cheek and gums. If your child won't or can't do that, carry it in *your* mouth. Finally, call a dentist without delay. Do *not* attempt to clean or scrub the tooth.

Electrical shock. The first order of business: Look out for yourself. If the child is in a puddle of water near a downed high-tension wire, for example, and you try to rescue him, you could be the second victim. The second order of business: Get emergency medical assistance immediately. If the child is not breathing, someone may have to breathe for him, but don't you do it unless you've been trained in first aid or cardiopulmonary resuscitation (CPR).

Eye injuries. More than 60,000 children suffer eye injuries every year, according to the National Society to Prevent Blindness. Many of these injuries are potentially very serious and could result in loss of vision. Here's what to do for the most common eye injuries.

Help for the Choking Child

The parents of younger children, in particular, need to be on their guard against choking. According to a nationwide study, inhalation of food or foreign objects causes 66 to 77 deaths annually in children under age ten.

Important: *Experts recommend that you seek emergency assistance if the following methods don't produce prompt results. It's also important to have a doctor examine the child after the object is removed.*

For infants under one year. Drape the child over one arm and administer four blows to the back, between the shoulder blades, with the heel of your palm. If these do not succeed in jarring the object loose, turn the baby over and give him four upward thrusts midway between his nipples, using the index and second finger of your hand. Be gentle. If the object is still stuck, go back to back blows, then chest thrusts, and so on, until the object is removed.

For children one year and older. Stand or kneel behind the child, bending the child's body forward from the waist, over one arm. Roll your free hand into a fist and place it, thumb side in, midway between the child's navel and the bottom tip of the breastbone. Administer four quick upward thrusts. If it doesn't work the first time, try it again.

If your child is hit in the eye, put that beefsteak back in the freezer. Instead, apply cold compresses to the injured eye for 15 minutes every hour. This should keep the swelling down. If the skin around the eye becomes discolored—in other words, a black eye—or if vision is blurred, go to your local emergency room. Ophthalmologists recommend that you not allow the child to blow his nose. And don't try to "make it better" by dabbing on any medication. You could make it worse.

For a chemical burn of the eye, hold the eyelids open and *gently* flush the eye with cold water continuously for 15 minutes. Don't use an eyewash and don't cover the eye with a bandage. Go immediately to the emergency room and take along the product container—gasoline, hairspray or whatever chemical caused the burn.

If a foreign object gets into your child's eye, tell him to blink his eyes. The resulting tears may wash out the offending particle. Do not allow him to rub his eyes. Gently lift the upper eyelid and pull it down over the lower eyelid. The lashes also may force the object out.

For cuts or punctures of the eye, forget direct pressure. If an eye is cut or punctured, you should *not* do anything to increase the pressure. You can apply a loose bandage with a clean dressing. Don't wash out the eye and, if something is stuck in the eye, do *not* try to remove it. Get emergency assistance immediately.

Foreign object in the nose or ear. This could be a potentially serious emergency. First aid, in this case, includes a couple of "don'ts" and a "do." Don't try to remove the object. Don't allow the child to slap the side of his head in an attempt to dislodge an object from his ear. And do call your physician or get the child to the hospital without delay.

High fever. This could become a serious medical emergency. If your child is under two years of age, contact a physician promptly if the child's temperature is unexplained or exceeds 104°F. This could be an indication of meningitis or other dangerous infections. Although a temperature of 104°F is not as critical for a child older than two, a physician should still be contacted.

Poisoning. Before you do anything else, call your local or regional poison information center. According to George C. Rodgers, Jr., M.D., associate professor of pediatrics at the University of Louisville, "They can give you the appropriate information."

Much has been said in the past about the value of syrup of ipecac, a substance used to induce vomiting, but vomiting isn't always necessary. Sometimes it can worsen an already bad situation.

"There are certain substances, like corrosives or petroleum products, that should not be brought back up," says Dr. Rodgers. "But a good poison center will prevent an awful lot of these unnecessary emergencies."

If you call the poison control center and they tell you to induce vomiting, you can use liquid dishwashing detergent—two tablespoons, followed by a glass of water—if you don't have ipecac on hand, says Dr. Rodgers. But, he adds, ipecac is much preferred. You should have one bottle on hand for each child under age five.

Sprained ankle. Unless you're an orthopedic surgeon—and sometimes not even then—you might not be able to tell what's sprained and what's broken. Elevate the injured ankle and take the child to the hospital. *Do not* have the child walk on the injured part. That's an old wives' tale, and a lame one, at that.

Index